Emergency Medicine and Trauma

Edited by Ozgur Karcioglu and Müge Günalp Eneyli

Published in London, United Kingdom

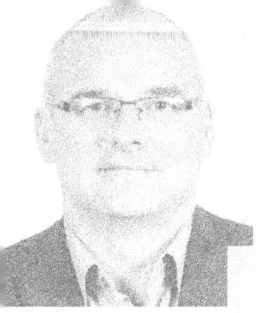
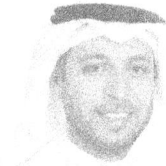
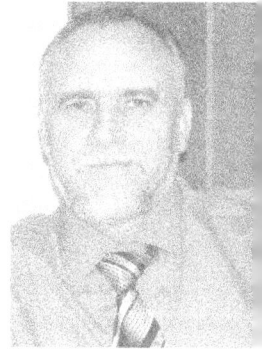
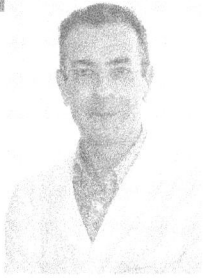
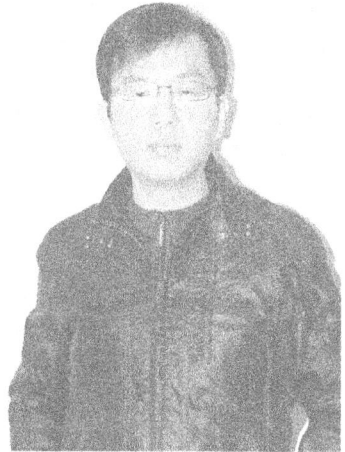
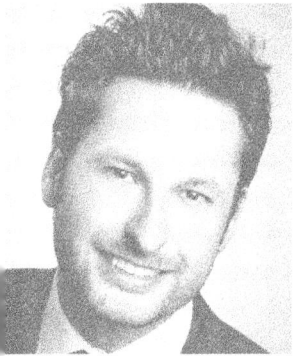
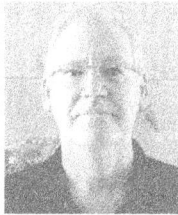

IntechOpen

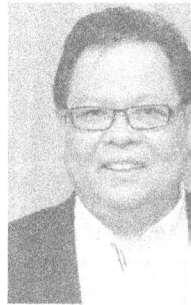
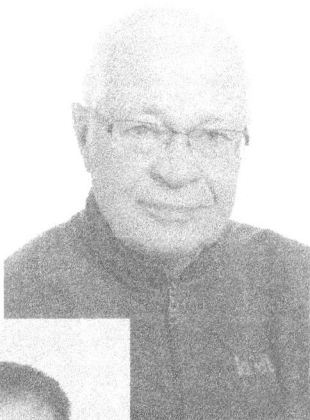
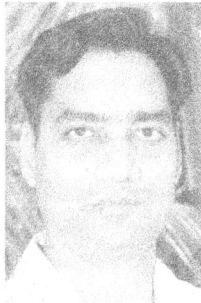
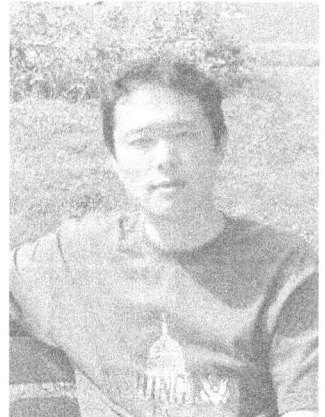
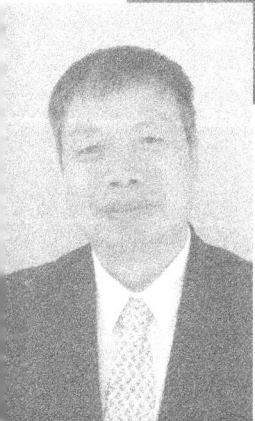
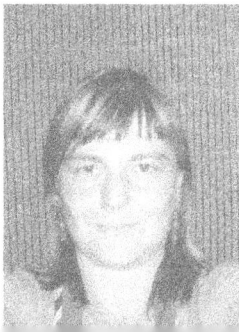

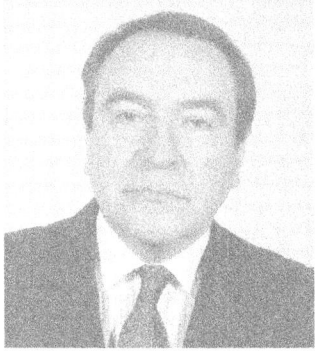

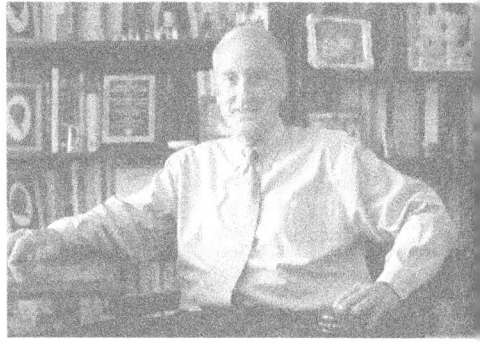

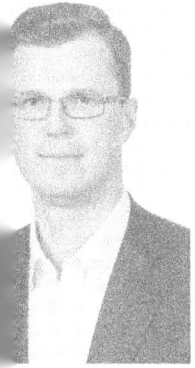

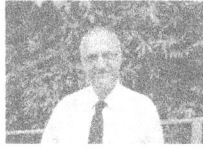

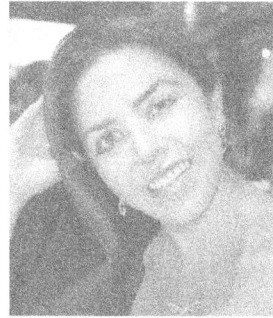

Supporting open minds since 2005

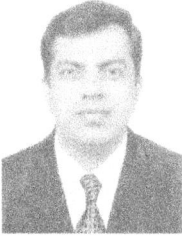

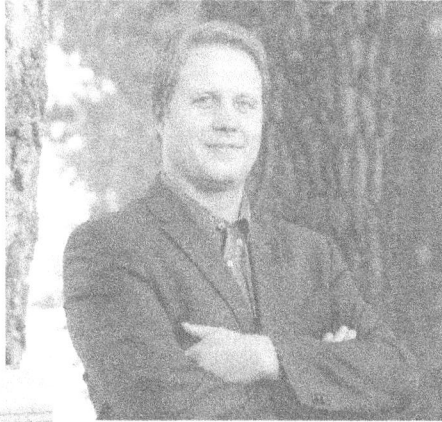

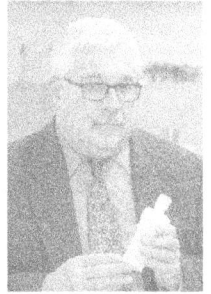

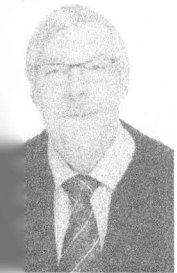

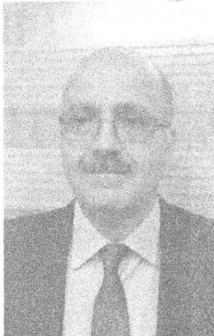

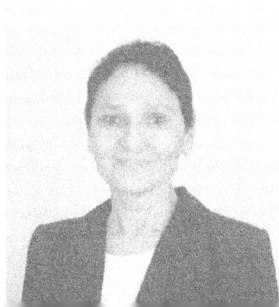

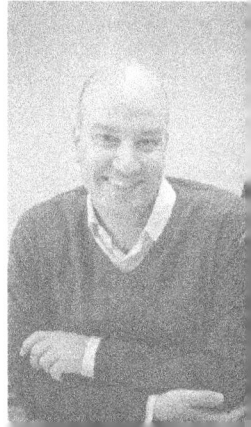

Emergency Medicine and Trauma
http://dx.doi.org/10.5772/intechopen.77738
Edited by Ozgur Karcioglu and Müge Günalp Eneyli

Contributors
Enoch F. Sam, David K Blay, Samuel Antwi, Constance Anarfi, Juliet Adoma Asum, Abdulnasir Al-Jazairi, Fran Laurie, TJ FitzGerald, Peter Lee, Matthew Iandoli, Ameer L. Elaimy, James Shen, Alexander Lukez, Lakshmi Shanmugham, Beth Herrick, Jonathan Glanzman, David Goff, Maryann Bishop-Jodoin, Rebeca Astorga Veganzones, Carmen Diana Cimpoesu, Tudor Ovidiu Popa, Paul Lucian Nedelea, Krzysztof Szaniewski, Tomasz Byrczek, Tomasz Sikora

Notice
Statements and opinions expressed in the chapters are these of the individual contributors and not necessarily those of the editors or publisher. No responsibility is accepted for the accuracy of information contained in the published chapters. The publisher assumes no responsibility for any damage or injury to persons or property arising out of the use of any materials, instructions, methods or ideas contained in the book.

First published in London, United Kingdom, 2019 by IntechOpen
IntechOpen is the global imprint of INTECHOPEN LIMITED, registered in England and Wales, registration number: 11086078, The Shard, 25th floor, 32 London Bridge Street London, SE19SG – United Kingdom
Printed in Croatia

British Library Cataloguing-in-Publication Data
A catalogue record for this book is available from the British Library

Additional hard and PDF copies can be obtained from orders@intechopen.com

Emergency Medicine and Trauma
Edited by Ozgur Karcioglu and Müge Günalp Eneyli
p. cm.
Print ISBN 978-1-78985-093-2
Online ISBN 978-1-78985-094-9
eBook (PDF) ISBN 978-1-83962-231-1

We are IntechOpen,
the world's leading publisher of
Open Access books
Built by scientists, for scientists

4,300+
Open access books available

116,000+
International authors and editors

130M+
Downloads

151
Countries delivered to

Our authors are among the

Top 1%
most cited scientists

12.2%
Contributors from top 500 universities

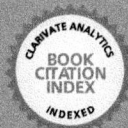

Interested in publishing with us?
Contact book.department@intechopen.com

Numbers displayed above are based on latest data collected.
For more information visit www.intechopen.com

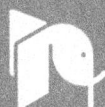

Meet the editors

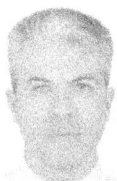

Dr. Karcioglu graduated from his residency in Dokuz Eylul University Medical School, Department of Emergency Medicine, Turkey, in 1998. He attended the "International Emergency Medicine" Fellowship in PennState University (2005). He is now the Chair of the Department of Emergency Medicine, Istanbul Education and Research Hospital.

Since 1995, he has served as a founder and board member of the Emergency Medical Association of Turkey. He has had around 130 articles published in scientific journals, and has contributed in five books as an editor and authored 35 chapters. Recently, he published the books Trauma Surgery and Poisoning in the Modern World with the collaboration of IntechOpen. He is also an instructor of the Advanced Cardiac Life Support Course.

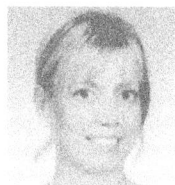

Dr. Günalp finished her residency in March 2004 at the Hacettepe University School of Medicine. She has been working as a clinical instructor in the Department of Emergency Medicine, University of Ankara, since. She has participated in emergency trauma care courses as an instructor since 2004. She also organized an advanced cardiac life support course in Turkey as a director between 2009 and 2012. At Ankara University School's Department of Emergency Medicine she prepared a project to the EU called "Improving the Research Potential of Medical School of Ankara University on Trauma Management System" for the Seventh Framework Programme (FP7) Regpot-2008-1. She also participated in this project as project manager. She participated in a core instructor course and became a BLS and ACLS instructor.

Contents

Preface

Rates of traumatic incidences have increased throughout the world. Economic burden and healthcare costs are also on the rise, with morbidity and mortality rates heightened unacceptably, especially in the developing countries. This trend can be easily attributed to a recent upsurge in terrorist assaults, warfare in general (including individual arming), disasters, and mass-transportation accidents. In response, healthcare personnel directly in charge of trauma management are pressurized to evaluate, diagnose, treat, and stabilize patients who have been exposed to some type of physical traumatic injury, as well as associated psychological and sociological suffering. Trauma resuscitation should comprise a collaboration of emergency medicine, surgical disciplines, intensive care medicine, and other ancillary services of the healthcare system. Trauma management is not confined to a "technical repair" of the injuries specific to body parts, but encompasses an integrative approach of resuscitation, restoration of the victim's homeostasis, and physiological and psychological support for the general welfare of both the individual and the community, which comprise the theme of this book. This book is intended to cover important aspects of trauma diagnosis and management of resultant injuries.

MD, FEMAT Ozgur Karcioglu
Professor,
Department of Emergency Medicine,
University of Health Sciences,
Istanbul Education and Research Hospital,
Fatih, Istanbul, Turkey

MD, FEMAT Müge Günalp Eneyli
Ankara University School of Medicine,
Turkey

Section 1

Prehospital Management of Trauma and Triage

Chapter 1

Pre-Hospital and Trauma Care to Road Traffic Accident Victims: Experiences of Residents Living along Accident-Prone Highways in Ghana

Enoch F. Sam, David K. Blay, Samuel Antwi,
Constance Anaafi and Juliet A. Adoma

Abstract

Road traffic accidents (RTAs) and associated injuries are a major public health problem in developing countries. The timely emergency pre-hospital care and subsequent transportation of accident victims to the health facility may help reduce the accident and injury outcomes. Available evidence suggests that RTA victims stand a greater chance of survival if attended to and cared for in a timely manner. This exploratory qualitative study set out to explore the experiences of residents of 12 communities along the Kasoa-Mankessim highway in Ghana (an accident-prone highway) in administering emergency pre-hospital care to RTA victims. We utilised data from a purposive sample of 80 respondents (i.e., people who have ever attended to RTA victims) from the communities through structured interview schedules. We found that the majority of the respondents had little knowledge and/or professional training in first-aid and emergency pre-hospital care to RTA victims. The skills and knowledge exhibited were gained through years of rescue services to RTA victims. The "scoop and run" method of first-aid care was predominant among the respondents. We recommend regular community member (layperson first responder) sensitisation and training on emergency pre-hospital care for RTA victims.

Keywords: road traffic accident victims, emergency pre-hospital care, layperson first responders, Kasoa-Mankessim highway, Ghana

1. Introduction

Road traffic accidents (RTAs) are associated with an estimated 1.25 million deaths globally each year with about 50 million others injured in the process [1]. The Ghanaian situation follows a similar trend. An estimated 1800 people are killed in road traffic accidents yearly with almost 14,500 others injured [2].

According to the WHO Global Burden of Disease project 2002, road traffic injuries (RTIs) are the 10th leading cause of death for all age groups globally, accounting for 1,183,492 deaths. More specifically, RTIs is the second and third leading cause of death for persons aged 5–29 years and 30–44 years, respectively [3, 4].

In low- and middle-income countries, RTIs constitute the ninth leading cause of death and the tenth leading cause of disability-adjusted life years (DALYs) [4, 5]. A number of factors account for the high RTIs in these countries including poorly maintained vehicles, inadequate traffic enforcement, inefficient pre-hospital emergency medical response and overburdened healthcare infrastructure [6]. As a result, about 80% of the injury deaths in these countries are said to occur in the pre-hospital setting [7].

Many of these injury deaths could be prevented with the timely arrival of competent emergency pre-hospital medical services at the accident scene [8, 9]. Timely emergency pre-hospital care to traffic accident victims at the accident scene and subsequent transportation to the health facility may reduce the probability of injury severity and deaths. Regarding injury severity and death, trauma experts consider the first 60 minutes (termed the "golden hour") after the injury occurred as the most important period to save lives. The risk of death or severe injury is believed to increase after this period [10].

Recently, the World Health Organisation has proposed training of layperson first responders as the first essential step in developing Emergency Medical Services systems in settings where the formal pre-hospital system is not available [6, 11]. This system has been found to be effective in reducing traffic accident-induced mortalities in most countries [5, 11–13]. A previous study revealed that about 51% of severely injured persons in Kumasi, Ghana died in a pre-hospital setting (cited in 7). This suggests that improving pre-hospital care to RTA victims is important to reduce "the mortality of critically injured roadway casualties" [7]. This stresses the urgency to establish layperson first responder care systems in Ghana (as proposed by the WHO) where formal pre-hospital care is inadequate. Pre-hospital care and post-crash intervention happen to be the focus of the fifth pillar of the UN Decade of Action of Road Safety 2011–2020 which aims to reduce the anticipated magnitude of RTAs and casualties [14].

1.1 Study objective

Given the important role of layperson first responders in the chances and quality of survival of RTA victims, this study explores the experiences of residents living along the Kasoa-Mankessim road network, an accident-prone road in Ghana, in administering emergency pre-hospital care to RTA victims. We explored their knowledge of pre-hospital first-aid and trauma care and the nature of the assistance they offer at accident scenes. The study results will expose the "pre-hospital trauma care knowledge and skill gaps" which can inform future training to facilitate safe handling and rescue of RTA victims in line with best practices. The remaining part of this paper proceeds as follows: Section 2 discusses the study methodology, while Sections 3–6 presents the study findings, discussion, study limitation and conclusion and implications for practice.

2. Methodology

We adopted a phenomenological research methodology [15] to explore and provide an in-depth description of participants' experiences/encounters with pre-hospital care for road traffic accident victims on the Kasoa-Mankessim highway (**Figure 1**) in the central region of Ghana. This highway is a segment of the Accra-Cape Coast road network. The entire road network is classified as a national route 1 (N1) road and also forms part of the Trans-West African Highway network.

The Kasoa-Mankessim section is a single two-lane carriageway (31.1 km in length; 7.3 m wide with 2.5 m shoulders on both sides). The road's posted speed

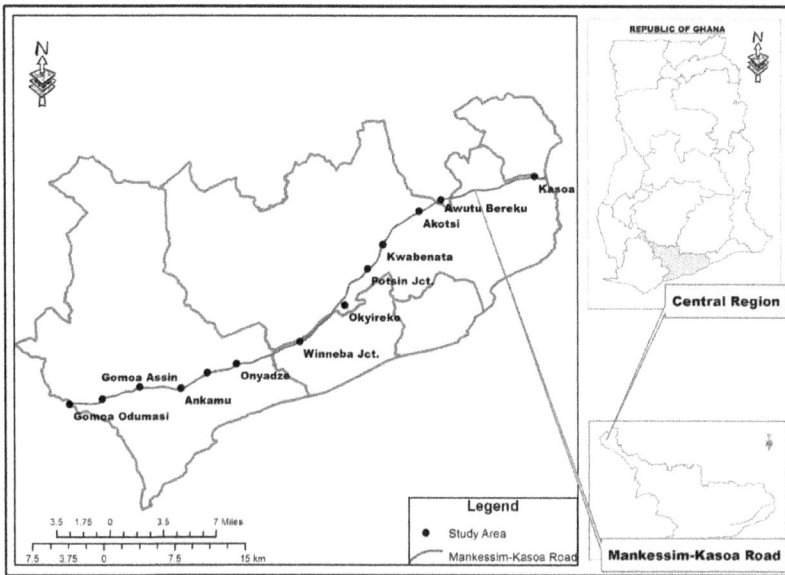

Figure 1.
Map of the study areas and road network.

is between 50 and 100 kph with a weighted average annual daily traffic volume of 9661 vehicles per day. The road links many settlements in the region to Accra, the national capital [16]. There are 11 'police-identified blackspots' on the road network namely Brigade, Galilea, Amanfrom, Potsin Junction, Budumburam, Okyereko Junction, Adawuku, Bible College Area, Tipper Junction, Awutu Beraku and Gomoa Buduatta Junction. These black spots are characterised by dangerous curves, slippery steeps, narrow bridges and undulating surfaces. For the year 2014 alone, 631 RTAs (i.e., 90 fatal, 137 serious, 158 slight and 246 property-damage-only accidents)[1] were recorded on the entire Accra-Cape Coast road network associated with 696 casualties (119 killed, 241 serious and 336 slight injuries). These figures translate into 4.5 accidents per kilometre and 4.9 casualties per kilometre [17].

2.1 Procedure

Prior to data collection (interviews), we carried out a reconnaissance visit to the selected communities. Our aim was to introduce the study to the community stakeholders, familiarise ourselves with the terrain, and pre-select and schedule interview appointments with potential respondents. At the data collection stage, we employed a mix of non-probability sampling techniques (i.e., purposive, convenient and snowball sampling techniques) in selecting the study participants and communities. Our study comprised of 80 purposive samples from 12 conveniently sampled communities/settlements (mostly blackspots) along the Kasoa-Mankessim road network (the communities are indicated in **Figure 1**). To be eligible to participate in the study, a person ought to have first-hand-on-the-spot experience assisting RTA victims on this road segment. At some stages of the data collection, we employed

---

[1] Fatal accident is here defined as an accident where at least one casualty dies of injuries sustained within 30 days of occurrence; serious injury accidents involve at least one casualty detained in hospital as an in-patient for more than 24 hours; slight injury accident is minor requiring at most first-aid attention for the casualties.

the snowball sampling technique to sample other eligible participants from our initial contacts. On average, we interviewed six persons in each community lasting nearly 15 minutes from March to April 2017.

2.2 Analysis

Data coding and analysis were done in stages. At the first stage, we produced a transcript of each interview in English (participants gave consent to the audio recording of the interviews) and loaded into the Atlas.ti 7.0 software. At the second stage, we conducted inductive data coding and analysis using open and *In Vivo* coding (to 'honour' participant's voice and to ground the analysis from their unique experiences and perspectives) [18]. Lastly, we conducted a thematic analysis of the data, resulting in two main themes namely, knowledge of pre-hospital care for road traffic accident victims and the nature of assistance offered to the accident victims.

3. Findings

Our sample was mainly males (83.7%) over 30 years old (53.8%) and mostly Junior High school graduates (43.7%) **Table 1**. Study sample characteristics (*n* = 80).

From our interviews, we gathered that at least an accident occurs every month on this road as evidenced by the quotes below. Interestingly, 2 days to the interviews, an accident occurred around Okyereko (one of the selected communities) as recounted by this respondent:

> *A sprinter bus had an accident just in front of our house 2 days ago (Male, 42 years, Okyereko).*

> *Yes, I have witnessed a number of road accidents on this highway. I can count about six of them and the last one I witnessed, 14 people died. This happened 2 weeks ago (Male, 29 years, Apam junction).*

> *On this road, almost every month we hear of road accidents. The last one I witnessed was about 3 weeks ago where everyone on board the vehicle died. I personally have witnessed more than seven accidents on this road and heard of uncountable others (Male, 33 years, Gomoa Mprumem).*

The accident-prone nature of this highway is depicted by the number of cautionary billboards planted close to previous accident spots. On each billboard, the number of people killed in a particular accident at a spot is indicated as shown in **Figure 2**.

Below, we present the study findings based on the themes and supported by relevant quotes from the transcript.

3.1 Knowledge of pre-hospital care for RTA victims

As it is customary for residents along the highway to attend to RTA victims in the event of accidents, we sought to explore their knowledge of some basic pre-hospital emergency care for RTA victims. Generally, we assessed respondents' knowledge of care for victims bleeding, recovery position for victims with fracture (broken bones) and basic airway control in unconscious persons.

Generally, we noted that the majority of the participants have no practical training in pre-hospital care for RTA victims. For those who have received some

Variable		N	%
Sex	Male	67	83.7
	Female	13	16.3
Age	18–25 years	17	21.2
	26–30 years	20	25.0
	Above 30 years	43	53.8
Education (attained)	Non-formal	7	8.7
	Junior High	35	43.7
	Senior High	27	33.7
	Tertiary	11	13.7
Total		80	100

Table 1.
Study sample (n = 80).

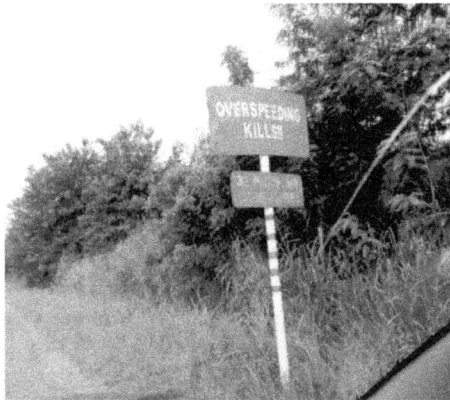

Figure 2.
Billboard indicating previous accidents on some spots on the highway.

training (n = 16 or 20%), they claimed it was just talk-based with a little demonstration. The rest acquired appreciable knowledge through years of rescue care for RTA victims.

> Yes. I remember one day, a group of people came here to talk to us about how we should handle accident victims. They said whenever we hear of a road accident, we should rush to the accident scene to help and try our best to call the Ambulance service and the Police. But it was mainly a talk show with little demonstration (Male, 32 years, Apam-junction).

Regarding victim recovery position(s) in the event of suspected fracture (broken bone), 20% of the participants (those with some training) rightly revealed that victim recovery position(s) depends on the nature of the injury sustained. They emphasised placing the victim on the ground as it is difficult to determine the nature of the injury sustained.

> Not all victims who are involved in road accidents sustain serious or severe injuries. So those victims who are not hurt or injured, some of them could stand and others

sit on the ground. But the severely injured victims should be placed on the floor with their backs to the ground (Male, 34 years, Apam-junction).

If the victim has a broken leg or hand, let the victim lie with the back to the ground. Usually, the position of the victim depends on the form of injury I suspect might have occurred (Male, 32 years, Apam-junction).

I think the casualty should be made to lie down at the back to get enough air because the casualty may be suffering from a spinal problem or a dislocated waist or leg and so allowing such a victim to sit or squat may result in other injuries (Male, 30 years, Potsin).

Yet, others, like this respondent, revealed:

I usually do not know the affected part of the victims, so my aim is to remove the victims from the car to be transported to the hospital (Male, 35 years, Gomoa Mprumem).

In case the victim is bleeding, most respondents (86%) demonstrated adequate knowledge of pre-hospital care including applying pressure to the affected area by pressing hard with the hands and subsequently applying local herbs or leaves and bandage to the bleeding part in order to stop or reduce bleeding (external compression for haemorrhage control).

I tear the victim's shirt and use it to bandage the affected part. This helps to reduce the bleeding to prevent loss of blood, even if there is a delay in transporting them to the hospital (Male, 34 years, Apam-junction).

I am a driver, so I usually use dusters from my car or the shirts of (male) victims to tie the bleeding part before I transport them to the hospital (Male, 37 years, Apam-junction).

It is evident from the interviews that bandaging or tying the bleeding area (haemorrhage control) is the common first aid most residents know of. However, others revealed different indigenous methods to stop bleeding.

For me, what I normally do is to look for leaves like "Acheampong" (a local herb) and I grind it on the road and apply it on the bleeding part to reduce the bleeding, or even at times I use plantain leaves, grind it and after that, I squeeze the water content on the bleeding part. Even though it hurts when the leaves are applied to injuries, but they help to reduce bleeding as soon as possible (Male, 35 years, Gomoa Mprumem).

Lastly, we also quizzed respondents on their knowledge on how to assist unresponsive RTA victims. About 27% of the respondents rightly suggested checking the victim's pulse and body movements to determine the chances of survival and shouting into the victim's ear to determine if the victim responds or not. Other participants also think because most unresponsive victims become short of breath, the best way to assist them is by placing them on the ground with the head tilted backwards to open the airway in the throat to enable the victim to take in more air (basic airway control in unconscious persons).

If the victim still breaths or the heart still beats, I put the victims in an open space to get more air. But if I cannot feel the heartbeat, I conclude that the victim is dead yet still we transport them to the hospital (Male, 35 years, Gomoa Mprumem).

In sum, we realised that the study respondents were more adequate in their knowledge of pre-hospital care for bleeding accident victim(s) than in the case of the recovery position for the victim(s) who suffer fracture (broken bones) or are unresponsive.

3.2 Nature of assistance offered to accident victims

Varied methods, mainly indigenous, are employed in saving RTA victims. **Figures 3–5** depict the kind of assistance community residents provide at accident scenes. We observed that the *"scoop and run"* method of pre-hospital care (which involves providing basic care at the trauma site and rushing the victim to a hospital) was the common practice among the respondents. Some respondents also call on the National Fire Service and the Ambulance Service to help. The quotes below illustrate the kind of assistance provided at accident scenes.

> *We have not been trained on how to administer first aid and also do not have what it takes to treat the accident victims, and so we usually arrange with an oncoming vehicle to transport them to the nearest hospital (Female, 34 years, Kwabenata).*

> *A taxi had an accident here 2 weeks ago and it caught fire. We all had to run to our homes to fetch water to quench the fire before we were able to remove the victims from the car (Male, 28 years, Kwabenata).*

However, the situation was different for those who had ever received some first-aid training:

> *I have received some training in first aid. As a taxi driver, I usually carry a first aid box in my car with the basic supplies. Anytime I witness an accident and the victims bleed, I wash the bleeding part with water and apply methylated spirit to the affected part(s) and subsequently put cotton wool and plaster to stop the bleed-ing. Shortly after, I transport the victims in my taxi to the hospital (Male, 38 years, Okyereko).*

Notwithstanding, we noted that the rescue efforts were often saddled with chal-lenges. The major challenge we noted was the lack of proper tools to cut open vehicles in order to bring out trapped victims. There was also the difficulty of rescuing victims in burning vehicles. Some respondents revealed sustaining burns and deep cuts by the broken glasses of the crashed vehicles in the process of rescuing victims.

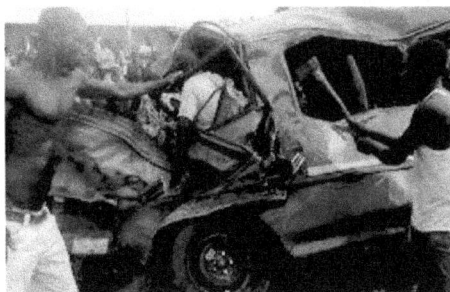

Figure 3.
Residents trying to rescue victims stacked in a vehicle.

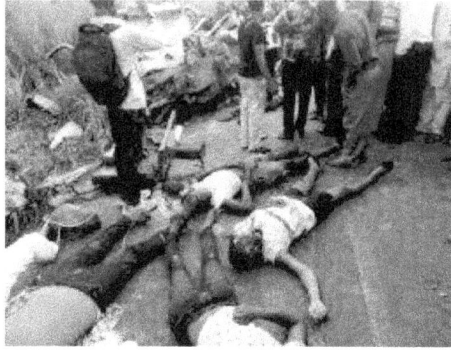

Figure 4.
RTA victims put at recovery position.

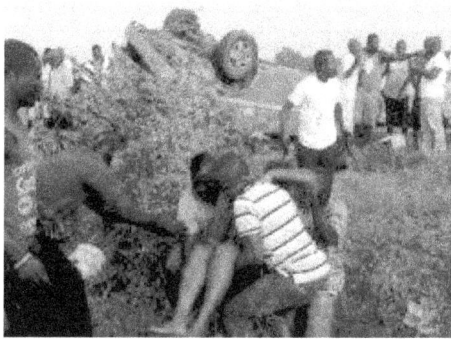

Figure 5.
Some community residents assisting RTA victims.

> *Our ability to rescue victims from crashed vehicles depend on the extent of damage to the vehicle. We lack the necessary equipment to cut open accident vehicles. Mostly, we use cutlass, axes and any available tool to cut the vehicle in order to get the victims out. We end up injuring ourselves in the process (Male, 35 years, Gomoa Mprumem).*

> *Whenever an accident occurs here and the vehicle catches fire, removing the victims becomes very difficult but because we want to help, we persist and end up sustaining injuries in the process (Male, 29 years, Kwabenata).*

4. Discussion

In this study, we sought to explore the experiences of residents of communities along the Kasoa-Mankessim highway in providing pre-hospital care to RTA victims. This knowledge is important to provide the basis for future training to ensure safe victim handling in line with international best practices. Recently, WHO has encouraged layperson first responder programmes as a basic step in the development of a functioning pre-hospital system [13]. Given that communities along accident-prone highways are normally the first people to come into contact with the RTA victims (first responders), the need to train them adequately cannot be overemphasised.

The current study found that there is a natural inclination to help RTA victims among the study respondents, yet only a handful of them have received proper pre-hospital training to facilitate safe victim handling and pre-hospital care in line with best practices. Of the 80 participants, only 20% had received some form of pre-hospital first-aid training, howbeit inadequate. In view of this, most participants had little knowledge in first aid care processes. As a consequence of the lack of training, participants had devised various strategies to assist RTA victims, which is likely to result in further injuries or even the death of victims.

It was also apparent that even though most of the respondents have not been trained in pre-hospital care to RTA victims, through continuous victim rescue efforts, they have gained some valuable experiences. However, respondents with some training exhibited appropriate knowledge of the pre-hospital procedures in the areas of our knowledge assessment consistent with previous findings [7, 12, 13].

Another important finding was that the scoop and run method of pre-hospital care [19] was common among the study participants. This could be explained by their little or no clinical (pre-hospital) know-how and appropriate tools and supplies to cater for RTA victims. This notwithstanding, available evidence suggests that the scoop and run method is effective in increasing the chance of victim survival in the event of serious injuries [19, 20]. Any delay to transport victims for definitive care decrease the chance of victim survival (which is time-critical) [20].

The study results further support the establishment of layperson first responder systems in pre-hospital deficient settings. Generally, the natural inclination to help RTA victims and the success of the programme in other countries, mostly in Africa makes this workable in our study areas [5, 11–13]. These studies demonstrate that trained layperson first responders retain and appropriately use their newly acquired knowledge and skills for societal good [7, 12].

5. Study limitation

It is noteworthy that similar studies were either quantitative in design or at best evaluation of the impact of a pre-hospital care or first-aid training course or a systematic review of the literature. Unlike these studies, our study was mainly qualitative and exploratory in nature and unique in its approach to exploring the knowledge of pre-hospital care for RTA victims. As a qualitative, exploratory study, it suffers from concerns with generalisability of the study findings to the population, a supposed problem associated with qualitative studies in general. However, the study findings are significant in their own right and provide a valuable first view of the processes residents of the named highway goes through to assist RTA victims which is important for further studies and intervention programmes.

6. Conclusion

Based on the study findings, we conclude that there is a general enthusiasm to assist RTA victims among the respondents and the communities, yet there are gaps in their knowledge of, and skills in pre-hospital care for RTA victims. The study findings thus suggest several courses of action in line with best practices.

To take advantage of community members' eagerness to assist RTA victims, the relevant stakeholders and policy-makers (Ghana Red Cross Society, National Ambulance, Ghana National Fire Service, and Ministry of Health) could undertake a couple of policy and practical actions toward ensuring efficient pre-hospital care for RTA victims.

The most obvious and immediate action involves implementing a functioning layperson first responder systems in the communities along the road network. As suggested in a previous study [7], persons (e.g., taxi drivers, community leaders) who are likely to chance upon and transport RTA victims could be the target of this layperson first responder training programmes. These persons should be equipped with the needed skills and first-aid kits/supplies to provide basic life support services pending definitive care as well as transport RTA victims to the nearest health facility. Periodic refresher training and incentives for the laypersons will ensure the sustainability of the system [6, 7]. As indicated earlier, this is an important and cost-effective step to developing formal emergency pre-hospital care systems [12]. Related to this is the urgent need to establish effective communication and transportation channels between the communities, the relevant stakeholders and health facilities.

It is also possible to utilise modern information and communication technology to send out messages to the relevant stakeholders in the event of RTAs. By the use of a global positioning system (GPS)-enabled devices, exact coordinates of accident locations could be sent to the national ambulance and other stakeholders for immediate deployment and assistance. For instance, the request for emergency service feature of the recently launched "*GhanaPost GPS App*" could be a useful system in this regard. This, however, implies that both community members and the relevant stakeholders should be trained to use it.

Last but not least, given that the driving population (motorists) are probably more likely to chance upon accident scenes, first-aid training/course could be made mandatory for motorists when obtaining a driving licence. This will ensure a well-equipped driving population who could promptly assist RTA victims should they chance upon an accident scene in the course of their journeys [20].

Acknowledgements

We are grateful to all persons who participated in the study. Without you, this study could not have come this far. We are also grateful to all stakeholders in the selected communities where we conducted interviews.

Conflict of interest

The authors declare no conflict of interest.

Author details

Enoch F. Sam*, David K. Blay, Samuel Antwi, Constance Anaafi
and Juliet A. Adoma
Department of Geography Education, University of Education, Winneba, Ghana

*Address all correspondence to: efsam@uew.edu.gh

References

[1] World Health Organization. Global Status Report on Road Safety 2015. Geneva: World Health Organisation; 2015. Available from: http://www.who.int/violence_injury_prevention/road_safety_status/2015/en/

[2] National Road Safety Committee. National Road Safety Strategy III (2011-2020). Accra: National Road Safety Commission; 2011

[3] Anthony DR. Promoting emergency medical care systems in the developing world: Weighing the costs. Global Public Health. 2011;**6**(8):906-913

[4] Krug EG, Sharma GK, Lozano R. The global burden of injuries. American Journal of Public Health. 2000;**90**(4):523-526

[5] Razzak JA, Kellermann AL. Emergency medical care in developing countries: Is it worthwhile? Bulletin of the World Health Organization. 2002;**80**:900-905

[6] Sasser S, Varghese M, Kellermann A, Lormand J-D. Prehospital Trauma Care Systems. Vol. 1. Geneva: World Health Organisation; 2005

[7] Tiska MA, Adu-Ampofo M, Boakye G, Tuuli L, Mock CN. A model of prehospital trauma training for laypersons devised in Africa. Emergency Medicine Journal. 2004;**21**(2):237-239

[8] Bigdeli M, Khorasani-Zavareh D, Mohammadi R. Pre-hospital care time intervals among victims of road traffic injuries in Iran. A cross-sectional study. BMC Public Health. 2010;**10**(1):406. Available from: http://bmcpublichealth.biomedcentral.com/articles/10.1186/1471-2458-10-406

[9] Peden M, Scurfield R, Sleet D, Mohan D, Hyder AA, Jarawan E, et al. World Report on Road Traffic Injury Prevention. Geneva: World Health Organisation; 2004. Available from: http://apps.who.int/iris/bitstream/10665/42871/1/9241562609.pdf

[10] Carr BG, Caplan JM, Pryor JP, Branas CC. A meta-analysis of prehospital care times for trauma. Prehospital Emergency Care. 2006;**10**(2):198-206. DOI: 10.1080/10903120500541324

[11] Callese TE, Richards CT, Shaw P, Schuetz SJ, Issa N, Paladino L, et al. Layperson trauma training in low- and middle-income countries: A review. Journal of Surgical Research. 2014;**190**(1):104-110. Available from: http://www.ncbi.nlm.nih.gov/pubmed/24746252

[12] Jayaraman S, Mabweijano JR, Lipnick MS, Cadwell N, Miyamoto J, Wangoda R, et al. First things first: Effectiveness and scalability of a basic prehospital trauma care program for lay first-responders in Kampala, Uganda. PLoS ONE. 2009;**4**(9):1-7

[13] Geduld H, Wallis L. Taxi driver training in Madagascar: The first step in developing a functioning prehospital emergency care system. Emergency Medicine Journal. 2011;**28**(9):794-796

[14] United Nations. Global Plan for the Decade of Action for Road Safety 2011-2020. Geneva: WHO; 2011. p. 25. Available from: http://scholar.google.com/scholar?hl=en&btnG=Search&q=intitle:Global+Plan+for+the+Decade+of+Action+for+Road+Safety+2011-2020#0

[15] Gray DE. Doing Research in the Real World. UK: Sage Publications; 2004

[16] Sam EF, Akansor J, Agyemang W. Understanding road traffic risks from the street hawker's perspective. International Journal of Injury Control

and Safety Promotion. 2019;**26**(1):92-98. Available from: http://www.tandfonline.com/action/journalInformation?journalCode=nics20

[17] National Road Safety Commission. Road Traffic Crashes in Ghana. Accra: National Road Safety Commission; 2014

[18] Saldana J. The Coding Manual for Qualitative Researchers. London, UK: Sage Publications Ltd; 2009. xii, 410 p

[19] Taran S. The scoop and run method of pre-clinical care for trauma victims. McGill Journal of Medicine. 2009;**12**(2):73-75. Available from: http://www.pubmedcentral.nih.gov/articlerender.fcgi?artid=2997263&tool=pmcentrez&rendertype=abstract

[20] Elvik R, Vaa T, Høye A, Sorensen M. The Handbook of Road Safety Measures. Bingley, UK: Emerald Group Publishing Limited; 2009. p. 1137

Chapter 2

Triage

Abdulnasir F.H. Aljazairi

Abstract

During austere conditions when there is a large demand on healthcare services and the resources are limited for different reasons, there should be a special way of managing patients and victims in order to make the most benefit to the community. Trial of first come, first served will lead to losing most of the seriously injured patients because they will reach late if they reached a healthcare facility. In addition, day-to-day work protocols with full resources also are not the optimum to offer for the whole community during a major incident. Triage has been created and evolved in military medical services to face mass casualty with limited resources and then transferred to civilian life to deal with mass casualty incidents. Applying triage to patients created some interference with medical bioethics if those applied on individual bases, but if applied in the whole picture of state or country, we can understand its rations.

Keywords: military triage, major incident, disaster, bioethics, sorting, emergency department triage

1. Introduction

God created human beings and honored them over other creatures; therefore, keeping life is one of utmost urges. This urge to save lives is challenged in time of major incidents when patients' needs are exceeding care resources. Moreover, with the increase in global population and escalation in the costs of healthcare, more patients are visiting emergency departments (EDs) all over the world to cut expenses and bypass remote appointments. Most EDs today adopt a triage system to prioritize patients who need urgent care.

2. Definition

2.1 Linguistic definition

"The process of determining the most important people or things from amongst a large number that require attention" [1].

2.2 In medical use

It is the sorting of victims by giving them grade to prioritize them for treatment and transportation in order to maximize the number of survivors in major incidents and war victims [2]. According to the assigned grade, patients will have their priority in attending by healthcare givers, investigations, and operation rooms.

The term triage is similar to "rationing" and "allocation" which is practiced on a daily basis in every field. For the term triage to be applied for a situation, there are three prerequisites that must be fulfilled:

1. There is shortage of resources in comparison to the needs.

2. There should be a system set to triage by the health body or facility.

3. Trained health personnel should do the triage [3].

3. History of triage

Triage started as war time medical effort driven by the increased number of wounded and shortage of resources. In addition the need for manpower during wars affected the priorities in triage in some armies.

It is believed that the first time triage used in military medicine to prioritize treatment for the wounded was by Baron Dominque Jean Larry (8 July 1766–25 July 1842). He made rules that the wounded are treated by the severity of their clinical conditions regardless of the rank; even enemies were treated in the same way [4].

The next milestone in triage was attributed to British rear admiral John Crawford Wilson (1834–4 July 1885) [5]. He differentiated between the severity levels of the wounded; he wrote in his book *Outlines of Naval Surgery*: "If a case should be hopeless, or the man apparently dying, an operation then would be useless" [6]. He was sorting wounded soldiers into three categories: slight, serious, and fatal. This was the base for further division in triage system by creation of the expectant zone. In the triage system created by Dominique, all serious cases are treated in the same level.

Triage in the American civil war was depending on the first-come, first-served basis regardless of the severity, salvageability, or best use of limited resources [3].

The World War I with the development of more lethal weapons like machine guns and chemical gases with a large number of wounds that could be treated pushed the military surgeons to apply and refine triage protocols. This has led to the concept of "The greatest good of the greatest number." This is the rule for triage practiced in military and civilian life during major incidents now [7]. This rule means that at time of limited resources and facing huge demand, some patients can be saved if long time and large amount of resources devote to them, but this will not be done. The reason to not offering help to those patients is that we can save much more number of wounded patients (who are less critical) using the same resources during the same time. We may save 10 patients instead of one. The pressure of escalating numbers of wounded soldiers with limited fighters in the battles made some health strategic planners in the armies to give higher priorities to patients that can be treated and sent back to front war lines rapidly over seriously injured patients that need urgent intervention for long duration. Winslow listed the two objectives of triage as "1st, conservation of manpower; 2nd, the conservation of the interest of the sick and wounded" [8].

In the World War II, the weapons were more developed with the introduction of tanks and air forces. On the other hand, medications and health services improved. The health strategic planners still concentrate on supporting the troops. They direct resources for soldiers who are able to fight rather than injured or diseased ones.

With the improvement of transportation and less dependence on the manpower in modern wars, it is rarely nowadays needed to leave somebody without treatment for the sake of others. The triage decision now is to which facility best transfer the patient and what is the optimum method of transportation.

4. Moral and ethical issues in triage

Health system ethics has been developing and improving since the eighteenth century by the First Geneva Conventions (1859) and Nuremberg Act [9]. In 1979, Beauchamp and Childress published their book *Principles of Biomedical Ethics* [10]. They put four main principles which are:

1. Respect of autonomy

2. Beneficence

3. Non-maleficence

4. Justice

4.1 Requirements for a triage system

To have a triage system, there are three requirements to be fulfilled:

A. There should be shortage of resources in comparison to the need.

B. There should be a system set by health authority to be used in such circumstances (point A).

C. There are personnel trained on the system who will implement it.

   If there is no shortage, then no need to use triage, but for every patient, the health facility will do its best to treat the patient.

   A triage system should be set by the health authority or facility administration to be followed by anyone doing this task. The aim of this step is to look for the benefit of the community and the population as a whole and not to just part of it.

D. Trained personnel to practice the triage to ensure the justice and prevent personal preference.

During major incidents, there are situations in which the triage officer should take some decisions that may be hard and not in the best interest of some patients. The decisions made by the planners in the First and Second World Wars and before are made not by patients' will or his best interest and benefit. Below is the discussion of the principles one by one:

1. Respect of autonomy: During a normal life, this is the first patient's right. No intervention should be done unless the patient understands the issue fully and accepts it. For this reason, the informed consent is needed to be signed by the patient. In time of major incidents with a large number of patients present, there should be prioritization of patients according to system agreed upon by the hospital or health authority. In time of major incidents, absolute knowledge of the whole community needs is predominant over individual liberty. It is sure

that some people will not be happy with delaying them regardless of their presentation time or their degree of severity.

2. Beneficence: In 1964, the World Medical Association (WMA) developed the Declaration of Helsinki as a set of ethical principles for experimentation on human beings. The declaration strongly emphasizes *(a)* that the concern for the interests of the subject must always prevail over the interests of science and society and *(b)* that ethical considerations must always take precedence over laws and regulations. Those principles cannot be applied during disaster conditions. The overall benefit to the community should overrule the personal benefit, and the concept of "maximum benefit to maximum number" should be used to maximize community benefit and welfare.

Later in the chapter, there is a section regarding exceptions to the general rules.

3. Non-maleficence: Non-maleficence means doing non-harming or inflicting the least harm possible to reach a beneficial outcome [11]. In this meaning trying to save as much as possible of the community can explain depriving some patients from treatment or delay them until suitable time and resources are available. In this issue we may not consider all people as the same, for example, if there is a healthcare giver and a fighter that are wounded, then we should not count each as one person, because when the healthcare giver is treated, he will help in saving the other.

4. Justice: In justice we mean that each patient should take what he needs and no one should be disadvantaged or deprived from treatment. People may misunderstand the meaning well and have high expectations to treat all patients as the highest-priority patient. To explain this we should differentiate between *equality* and *justice*. The first one means that everybody should receive the same amount. For example, a patient with fracture can wait for days, while the unconscious patient with multiple injuries needs rapid assessment and a full management plan rapidly implemented. This is justice; each patient will take time and resources according to the severity of the condition.

5. Ownership of resources is challenged in time of major incidents, and the hospital should accept and treat any patient involved in the incident (according to the plan) [3].

5. Special circumstances in triage

Although triage depends mainly on patients' injury severity, there are conditions which oblige the officer to modify his triage decision or in austere condition to decide to whom priority of care is given. The triage officer should look to the whole picture of the community, putting in his mind the aims at that particular time he is doing it and the full resources in addition to the type of patients he is dealing with. The following are examples of special conditions which need special care and by no means are they exhaustive:

A. Children: Dealing with children is sensitive not only from the emotional side but also the practical side. Children have more expected life span than old people, and in time of limited resources with the equality of other factors, priority should be given to children for the sake of the community.

B. Pregnant women: In dealing with pregnant women, we are dealing with two lives; therefore, they have double importance and should take priority.

C. Emergency services personnel: All those personnel should not be counted as one person; if we give them priority and save them, they will help in saving more lives. We give them the value of the expected number of lives they may save. In addition taking care of someone injured rapidly will encourage other to put all their efforts, knowing that their colleagues will treat them in high priority if they are injured, and this will improve the quality of care given to all patients.

D. People with special skills or knowledge or with special importance: There are some people who possess some special knowledge and skills or have some special importance to the country. Those should also get special treatment and priority. This will need confirmation of their status and priority from local or national authority to recognize them during major incidents.

E. The surrounding circumstance: If there is a critical need to manpower like in war condition, for example, then the triage officer may make the highest priority to simple cases that can be treated with minimal resources and time and go back to combat area. Another example is facing floods and waiting for central help, until extra help reaches them, and there is a desperate need for all hands even the slightly wounded; otherwise, the whole area and local community will have grave outcomes.

F. Combination of the abovementioned conditions needs the triaging officer to put his priority at that single moment.

6. Common triage systems

We can divide triage systems into several categories:

1. Military triage system

2. Major incidents in civilian life

3. Emergency department triage system which is used for managing patients on a daily basis

1. **Military triage system**: The military triage differs from civilian life because in many occasions there is chaos and many of the infrastructures are not present or destroyed by the combat. Another reason is that the troops are usually located outside the cities where there are no or small services and they need to build their own treatment and evacuation system. The healthcare in present time is provided to every wounded for two reasons. First, there is no dependence on manpower like previous battles, and, second, there is huge improvement in communication and transportation tools and equipment. Now every wounded soldier is treated, but the difference is in time and place.

2. **Major incidents in civilian life**: Civilian triage started around 200 years after the military one. The first triage system is simple triage and rapid treatment (START) which is a method used in the field to rapidly sort and prioritize patients during major incidents according to the severity of their injuries. It was developed in 1983 in California [12, 13]. Later there will be discussion of other systems that are developed later.

The triage systems used in military and major incidents "that occur in civilian life" are the same, and it will be discussed in combination. They differ in the infrastructures supporting each one, with clear overlap between them.

Table 1 shows some of scoring systems used to evaluate the severity of the injuries which is the base for triage.

There are different categories for triage in major incidents. They are the physiological and the anatomical methods.

Year introduced	Abbreviation	Name
1970	AIS	Abbreviated injury scale
1971	TI	Trauma index
1974	GCS	Glasgow Coma Scale
1974	TISS	Therapeutic intervention
1974	ISS	Injury severity score
1980	TI	Triage index
1980	TRISS	Trauma injury and severity score
1981	APACHE	Acute physiological and chronic health evaluation
1982	PGCS	Pediatric GCS
1987	PT	Pediatric trauma score
1987	OIS	Organ injury scale (AAST)
1988	PRISM	Pediatric risk of mortality score
1989	AP	Anatomical profile
1989	RTS	Revised trauma score
1989	T-RTS	Triage version of RTS
1990	ASCOT	A severity characterization of trauma
1994	UST	Uniform scoring system for trauma (Utstein style)
1994	APSC	Acute physiology score for children
1996	ICD-9-CM	ICD-9 clinical modification based on AIS and ISS
1996	TOXALSTM	Toxic advanced life support TM
1997	NISS	New ISS
2001	ASPTS	Age-specific pediatric trauma score
2002	PAAT	Pediatric age-adjusted TRISS
2003	START	Simple triage and rapid treatment
2003	JUMP-START	Pediatric version of START

The year input is the first time the system was introduced. Some has been updated later.

Table 1.
List of scoring systems [14].

The physiological systems are easily learned and need simple training; any health personnel can be trained and perform it. Moreover it can be reproduced easily and is a reliable method of following up the patient's condition. On the other hand, it is time-consuming and not suitable for incidents with a huge number of victims.

Anatomical systems of triage are fast and depend on visual recognition of injuries. These methods need a good amount of experience in injuries and when the patient needs surgery. It is difficult to reproduce the results as it is subjective and not objective. A very large number of victims is suitable for this type of triage.

After knowledge of the anatomical and physiological condition of patients, the triage officer needs to know the comorbidities to and other circumstances (discussed above in the section of special situations) to give the patient the final triage level.

The most common triage systems used in major incidents are as follows:

A. **Glasgow Coma Scale**: It is a scoring system used to evaluate the patients with coma or disturbed consciousness (**Table 2**). It was first described by Graham Teasdale and Bryan Jennett in 1974 and was used as a practical method to evaluate patients with brain injury and a good method to communicate the patient's condition between different healthcare providers or facilities. The findings use the scale guide initial decision-making and monitor trends in responsiveness that are important in signaling the need for new actions [15]. Each point will be given a number: the maximum score is (15) and means the patient is fully conscious, and the lowest is (3) which is clearly seriously injured. The reactions to be noticed are:

There are studies comparing the full GCS to the motor reaction alone. It is believed that motor response is better predictive of patients' condition than full GCS [16]. Recently the use of GCS in triage is objected because it is time-consuming and can be interpreted in different combinations for the same score [17].

B. **Simple triage and rapid treatment (START)**: It is currently widely used in the United States and many other countries. People can be easily trained on it and used to sort victims rapidly into four categories: red, yellow, green, and white (or black). It depends on the ability of the victim to walk and then give the green category. If the patient cannot walk and has any alteration in his level of consciousness or vital signs, then he is categorized as red. If there is no alteration, he will be yellow. If no breathing and unconscious, then he is considered dead (white). **Figure 1** shows the flowchart for START triage system [18].

C. **JumpSTART**: It is the pediatric version of the START system; the main difference is the trial with the child to do airway maneuver and short

Eyes		Verbal		Motor	
Spontaneous	4	Orientated	5	Obey commands	6
To sound	3	Confused	4	Localizing	5
To pressure	2	Words	3	Normal flexion	4
None	1	Sounds	2	Abnormal flexion	3
		None	1	Extension	2
				None	1

Table 2.
Glasgow Coma Scale (GCS). (glasgowcomascale.org) [15].

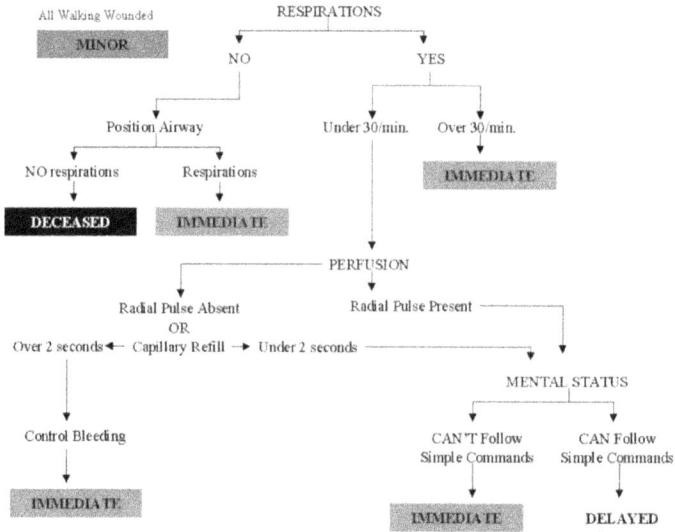

Figure 1.
Flowchart for START triage system [18].

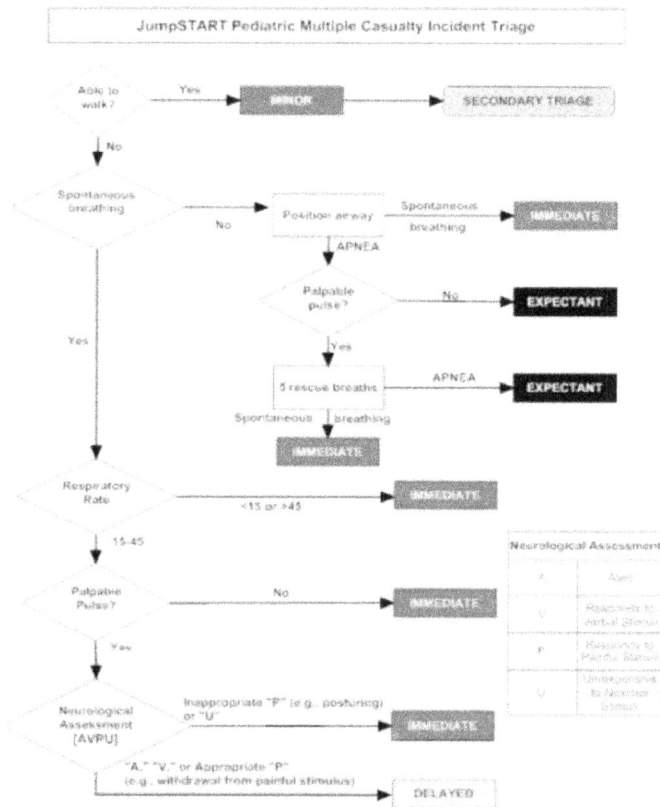

Figure 2.
Flow sheet for JumpSTART triage system [18].

resuscitation trial in the field before declaring death of the child. In addition to considering the change of heart rate in different age groups, **Figure 2** shows the flowchart for JumpSTART triage system.

D. **Triage-revised trauma score (T-RTS):** This system depends on physiological parameters of the patient at the time of evaluation. It is found to be a good indicator of the severity of the injury [19]. It depends on three physiological parameters which are (1) Glasgow Coma Score (GCS), (2) systolic blood pressure (BP), and (3) respiratory rate (RR). Each factor will be given a score, and then the scores of the three factors are summed: the more the score, the

STEP 1: calcurate the physiologic variables

A Respiratory rate, /min

	points
10-29	4
>29	3
6-9	2
1-5	1
0	0

B Systolic blood pressure, mmHg

	points
≥ 90	4
76-89	3
50-75	2
1-49	1
0	0

C Glasgow coma score

	points
13-15	4
9-12	3
6-8	2
4-5	1
3	0

$$TRTS = A + B + C$$

STEP 2: Assign a triage priority

TRTS	triage priority
1-10	Immediate
11	Urgent
12	Delayed
0	Dead

Step 1: Different variables in TRTS. Step 2: Interpretation of the results.

Table 3.
Triage-revised trauma score [19].

Categories and urgencies in the emergency triage system	
Category	Urgency of the condition
One	Patients in this category should be attended immediately when presented
Two	Patients will have priority and seen in the next doctor available. By passing que of patients present
Three	To place the patient's file at the front of the waiting list
Four	Wait for their que or may be advised to go to a primary health facility
Five	Discharged from emergency side and advised to visit the primary health facility

Table 4.
The five levels of triage in emergency department [21].

better the condition of the patient and vice versa. **Table 3** shows the different items in T-RTS and their interpretation.

There are several other systems, but they are used to assess and predict prognosis in trauma patients and not used for prioritizing them during response to major incidents.

3. **Emergency department triage systems**: The emergency department shares with the military life the inability to control the number and time of patients presented. With timeliness of the care and relative scarce of resources, in addition to the increase in the demand on beds and blocked access to other services, more patients are seeking medical care in emergency departments [20]. To make risk assessment of patient introduced to the ED and make the best benefit of the resources, a five-level triage system was introduced in Ipswich, Australia. This system was validated and adopted in several states in Australia and formed the base for different national systems in several countries in the world. The triage is done by experienced nurses, will give patients one of the five levels depending on the urgency of the conditions. **Table 4** shows the five levels in emergency department triage and the period allowed before attending the patient [21].

There are several triaging systems in different countries like the Manchester triage system which is widely used in the UK hospitals and the Canadian triage system (CTAS) and others, all using five levels and basically similar in sorting patients. There are minimal differences in the bench mark for the time frame each category should be seen within.

7. Wrong triage

With the rush and chaos occurring during response to major incidents, there are mistakes that may be committed by the triaging officer. Under-triage and over-triage are the wrong decisions that may occur:

1. **Under-triage**: It is defined as "A term of art referring to underestimating the urgency of the condition of a person arriving in A&E and not prioritizing his or her management over that of a patient with less urgent needs" [22]. It is a medical problem and may result is serious bad outcomes because it deprives a patient from the resources he/she needs. What is the level of acceptable risk of under-triage? The CDC puts the threshold as 20%, but in practice it is 35% [23].

If the validation depends on the injury severity score (ISS) and any patient with a score of >15 transferred to a hospital without trauma center, then the acceptable level is 5% [24]. It is found that patients with under-triage have less mortality rate than patients with right triage to the trauma centers because they have better GCS score, blood pressure, and base deficit [25].

2. **Over-triage**: A term of art referring to unintentionally overestimating the urgency of the condition of a person arriving in A&E (casualty) and prioritizing that person's management over that of a patient with more urgent needs [26]. This is a less risky medical mistake. Its effect is on the limited resources during a major incident in terms of human resources, stuff used, or space occupied, e.g., intensive care beds, CT scan, operating theater, etc.; due to its low risk to patients, it is agreed that 25–50% is accepted [25].

8. Summary

Triage is a key step in managing major incidents properly. It is not contradicting bioethics, but it is looking from a different focus to make the best to the whole community. It has no rigid rules, and the triage officer must look for different aspects of resources and patients' situation to make the best triage decision leading to most benefits for all.

Author details

Abdulnasir F.H. Aljazairi
Emergency Department, Hamad Medical Corporation, Qatar

*Address all correspondence to: ahuaidi@hamad.qa

IntechOpen

References

[1] Oxford dictionary. Available from: https://en.oxforddictionaries.com/definition/triage [Accessed: 1 March 2019]

[2] Triage (n.) in Merriam Webester dictionary. Retrieved from: https://www.merriam-webster.com/dictionary/triage [Accessed: 1 February 2019]

[3] http://scholar.google.com/scholar_url?url=https://www.researchgate.net/profile/Kenneth_Iserson/publication/262637907_Triage_Ethics-Part_1/links/0f3175384caa07fc8a000000.pdf&hl=ar&sa=X&scisig=AAGBfm1ChejVnHa5pPw72hFGiaDK2zyl2Q&nossl=1&oi=scholarr [Accessed: 1 March 2019]

[4] Nakao H, Ukai I, Kotani J. A review of the history of the origin of triage from a disaster medicine perspective. Acute Medicine & Surgery. 2017;**4**(4):379-384. DOI: 10.1002/ams2.293

[5] https://en.wikipedia.org/wiki/John_Wilson_(Royal_Navy_officer) [Accessed: 8 March 2019]

[6] John Wilson D. Outlines of Naval Surgery. Edinburgh: MACLACHLAN, STEWART & Co. p. 26. Available from: https://books.google.com.qa [Accessed: 8 March 2019]

[7] Keen WW. The Treatment of War Wounds (Classic Reprint). Forgotten Books; 2017. W. B. Saunders Company 1918. Available from: https://archive.org/details/treatmentofwarwo00keen/page/13 [Accessed: 3 April 2019]

[8] Manring MM, Hawk A, Calhoun JH, Andersen RC. Treatment of war wounds: A historical review. Clinical Orthopaedics and Related Research. 2009;**467**(8):2168-2191. DOI: 10.1007/s11999-009-0738-5. Available from: https://www.ncbi.nlm.nih.gov/pmc/articles/PMC2706344/ [Accessed: 3 April 2019]

[9] Bernd D, Tobias K, Stefan G, Peter B, Tanja G. Ethical aspects of triage. 2 VOJENSKÉ ZDRAVOTNICKÉ LISTY ROČNÍK LXXIX, 2010, č. P 77–82. Available from: https://www.mmsl.cz/pdfs/mms/2010/02/08.pdf [Accessed: 3 April 2019]

[10] Beauchamp TL. Childress JF: Principles of Biomedical Ethics. New York: Oxford University Press; 2009

[11] Sundean LJ, McGrath JM. Ethical considerations in the neonatal intensive care unit. Available from: https://www.medscape.com/viewarticle/811079_5 [Accessed: 10 March 2019

[12] Ciottone GR, Biddinger PD, Darling RG, et al. Ciottone's Disaster Medicine. Elsevier Health Sciences; 2015. Available from: https://books.google.com.qa/books?redir_esc=y&hl=ar&id=9cUMogEACAAJ&q=START+TRIAGE+SYSTEM#v=snippet&q=START%20TRIAGE%20SYSTEM&f=false [Accessed: 12 March 2019]

[13] Lee CH. Disaster and mass casualty triage. AMA Journal of Ethics. Virtual Mentor. 2010;**12**(6):466-470. DOI: 10.1001/virtualmentor.2010.12.6.cprl1-1006. Available from: https://journalofethics.ama-assn.org/article/disaster-and-mass-casualty-triage/2010-06 [Accessed: 4 April 2019]

[14] Wilson WC, Grande CM, Hoyt DB. Trauma, Emergency Resuscitation, Perioperative Anesthesia, Surgical Management. AMA Journal of Ethics. CRC Press; 2007. Available from: https://books.google.com.qa/books?id=6FPvBQAAQBAJ&pg=PA60&lpg=PA60&dq=%22Acute+physiological+and+chronic+health+Evaluation%22+triage&source=bl&ots=PO9hPZEU4x&sig=ACfU3U1bjru8o5_HzgmJI-mg9v-d2OZahg&hl=ar&sa=X&ved=2ahUKEwjC5IuapLLhAhXF8HMBHRkGAmQQ6

AEwA3oECAgQAQ#v=onepage&q=%22Acute%20physiological%20and%20chronic%20health%20Evaluation%22%20triage&f=false [Accessed: 2 April 2019]

[15] https://www.glasgowcomascale.org/what-is-gcs/ [Accessed: 15 March 2019]

[16] Healey C, Osler TM, Rogers FB, et al. Improving the Glasgow coma scale score: Motor score alone is a better predictor. The Journal of Trauma. 2003;**54**(4):671-678. Available from: https://insights.ovid.com/pubmed?pmid=12707528 [Accessed: 1 April 2019]

[17] Stratton SJ. Glasgow coma scale score in trauma triage: A measurement without meaning. Annals of Emergency Medicine. 2018;**72**(3):270-271. Available from: https://insights.ovid.com/crossref/00000566–201809000-00008?isFromRelatedArticle=Y [Accessed: 1 April 2019]

[18] Bazyar J, Farrokhi M, Khankeh H. Triage Systems in Mass Casualty Incidents and Disasters: A review study with a worldwide approach. Open Access Macedonian Journal of Medical Sciences. 2019;**7**(3):482-494. DOI: 10.3889/oamjms.2019.119. Available from: https://www.ncbi.nlm.nih.gov/pmc/articles/PMC6390156/ [Accessed: 1 April 2019]

[19] Lichtveld RA, Spijkers AT, Hoogendoorn JM, Panhuizen IF, Van der werken C. Triage revised trauma score change between first assessment and arrival at the hospital to predict mortality. International Journal of Emergency Medicine. 2008;**1**(1):21-26. Available from: https://www.ncbi.nlm.nih.gov/pmc/articles/PMC2536180/ [Accessed: 2 April 2019]

[20] Fitzgerald G, Jelinek GA, Scott D, Gerdtz MF. Emergency department triage revisited. Emergency Medicine Journal. 2010;**27**(2):86-92. Available

from: https://www.ncbi.nlm.nih.gov/pubmed/20156855 [Accessed: 2 April 2019]

[21] Hospital triage. NSW, Australia. Available from: https://www.health.nsw.gov.au/Hospitals/Going_To_hospital/Pages/triage.aspx [Accessed: 3 April 2019]

[22] Available from: https://medical-dictionary.thefreedictionary.com/undertriage [Accessed: 16 March 2019]

[23] Nishimoto T, Mukaigawa K, Tominaga S, et al. Serious injury prediction algorithm based on large-scale data and under-triage control. Accident; Analysis and Prevention. 2017;**98**:266-276. Available from: https://www.sciencedirect.com/science/article/pii/S000145751630358X [Accessed: 3 April 2019]

[24] Barsi C, Harris P, Menaik R, Reis NC, Munnangi S, Elfond M. Risk factors and mortality associated with undertriage at a level I safety-net trauma center: A retrospective study. Open Access Emergency Medicine. 2016;**8**:103-110. Available from: https://www.ncbi.nlm.nih.gov/pmc/articles/PMC5108619/ [Accessed: 3 April 2019]

[25] Davis JW, Dirks RC, Sue LP, Kaups KL. Attempting to validate the overtriage/undertriage matrix at a level I trauma center. Journal of Trauma and Acute Care Surgery. 2017;**83**(6):1173-1178. Available from: https://www.ncbi.nlm.nih.gov/pmc/articles/PMC5732627/ [Accessed: 16 March 2019]

[26] Retrieved from: https://medical-dictionary.thefreedictionary.com/overtriage [Accessed: 3 April 2019]

Chapter 3

Prehospital Emergency Care in Acute Trauma Conditions

Tudor Ovidiu Popa, Diana Carmen Cimpoesu
and Paul Lucian Nedelea

Abstract

It is well known at this moment that a systems and systematic approach to trauma care cases is ideal. The prehospital controversies of in-the-field care in trauma cases, resuscitation, and transport, ground or air, are still debated. The most controversial is rapid transport to definitive care ("scoop and run") versus field stabilization in trauma, which remains a topic of debate and resulted in great variability of prehospital policy. Emergency medical services, including ground and air transportation, significantly extend the reach of tertiary care facilities, leading to rapid transport of critically ill patients. Emergency medical services (EMS) providers are the first link to a trauma care system, and trauma triage made by EMS personnel is also a very important factor in a good outcome of trauma patients. The assessment of patient and the treatment delivered by the first medical crew could have a large impact over the clinical evolution and output of trauma patient; that way, it is necessary to apply a systematic approach in this pathology, guided by clear and simple-to-follow recommendations applied on the scene. Recent review of the literature on helicopter emergency medical services (HEMS) showed an overall benefit of 2.7 additional lives saved per 100 HEMS activations.

Keywords: trauma, primary assessment, trauma algorithm, prehospital care, HEMS, ground ambulance transfer

1. Introduction

Emergency management of a patient with multiple trauma is complex and takes place on several stages and successive levels, requiring a great deal of specialized forces and expertise, experience, and competence and carrying out a number of risks that crews have to know, consciously assume, and learn to control and avoid them.

Trauma is a consequence of an unexpected event, which appears sometime in plain health; that is why, one of the main goals is to return the patient to a level of function as close to preinjury as possible. The other goals of trauma patient management are to identify and treat first life-threatening injuries and to prevent exacerbation of existing injuries or the appearance of additional injuries [1–3].

We will present in this chapter the recommendation during primary assessment for trauma patients, treatment required in this point, and recommendation before and during transport.

There is a large consensus that the outcome for trauma patients is improved with a systematic, multispecialty, and interdisciplinary approach from prehospital and hospital care teams. The first approach in trauma patient will be different compared with the well-known approach applied to a nontraumatic patient, which includes anamnesis, medical history, clinical and paraclinical exams, a definitive diagnosis confirmed also by imagistic diagnosis, and follow-up after treatment.

The general principles for trauma patient management are as follows:

- Treat the greatest life-threatening injuries first.

- Definitive and complete paraclinical and imagistic diagnosis is not immediately important; there is enough to diagnose the presence of clinical signs.

- Time is very important ("trauma patients' golden hour," which emphasizes the importance of rapid sequences of diagnosis and treatment).

- Assess, intervene, and reassess [1, 2].

In prehospital, after the primary assessment and the beginning of therapeutic approach, the patient will be transported to the hospital to receive definitive treatment. The modes of transportation are represented by road or air transfer. The decision to use HEMS transfer depends on several important geographical, physiological, and pathological factors needed to be considered.

The transfer of a seriously injured patient by helicopter may be sometimes hazardous and transportation by road could be in some circumstances a better and safer option. Other factors, including the clinical skills and experience of the helicopter crews, also need to be considered. A good knowledge of the area, resources at and flight time duration to trauma center hospitals, and the location of the landing zones (if helipads exist or nearest landing sites) also need consideration. A detailed estimation of transport time from the scene to the hospital is required to assess if ground or air ambulance transfer will offer the fastest way of transport to hospital. [1–3].

When a helicopter is requested by a ground crew already on scene, helicopter crew preparation and flight times may delay transfer times further. So, considering all these factors, a ground ambulance transfer could be a faster mode of transport than secondary air ambulance transfer.

2. Primary assessment and management

The management of the patient with multiple trauma should be carried out more than for other types of urgency, under the concept of the "golden hour," referring to the first hour after the accident, during which the patient is advised to end up in a trauma center and receive definitive treatment. In this "golden hour," the first 10 min from the time of the accident is called "platinum minutes", precisely to highlight the importance in the traumatized patients' economy and implicitly in deciding their chance of survival.

This is the densest time interval at the scene of the accident, the interval that decides the percentage of "avoidable deaths" in the trauma [1–3].

Because in these cases time is crucial, a systematic approach that can be rapidly applied is essential. This approach, named primary or initial assessment, includes the following steps:

- Triage in case of multiple victims

- Primary assessment—ABCDE—with immediate therapeutic measures for patients with life-threatening injuries

- Consideration of the need for patient transfer to a more specialized medical center

- Secondary survey, which includes a complete physical exam, "head-to-toe," and patient medical history

- Continuous monitoring and reevaluation

- Definitive care

In this particularly complex gear, the chance of survival of a traumatized patient is also conditioned by the implementation of a specific "chain of survival," which is represented by the following links described in **Figure 1**.

Posttraumatic cardiac arrest produces a very high mortality, but in patients with the return to spontaneous circulation, the neurological status of the survivors seems to be much better than in other causes of cardiac arrest.

The response to posttraumatic cardiac arrest must be rapid and success depends on a well-established chain of survival, which includes advanced care in prehospital and transport to specialized trauma centers. Immediate resuscitation efforts in posttraumatic cardiac arrest are concentrated on the simultaneous treatment of reversible causes, which have priority over sternal compressions [1–3].

The periarrest condition is characterized by cardiovascular instability, hypotension, absence of peripheral pulse in nontraumatized areas, and a level of consciousness deteriorating without being due to the central nervous system. Untreated, this condition will progress to cardiac arrest.

Focused assessment with sonography in trauma (FAST ultrasound examination) can be helpful in diagnosis and management, but it should not delay resuscitation efforts [4].

It is vital that a medical cardiac arrest should not be attributed to a posttraumatic cardiac arrest and this must be treated under the universal ALS algorithm. Cardiac arrest or other causes of sudden loss of consciousness (e.g., hypoglycemia, stroke, and seizures) may be the cause of secondary traumatic effects [1–3].

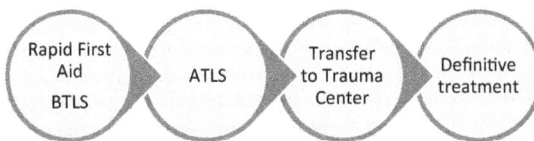

Figure 1.
Trauma chain of survival; BTLS, basic trauma life support; ATLS, advanced trauma life support.

2.1 Diagnosis

Diagnosis of the posttraumatic cardiac arrest is only clinical. The patient has agonistic respiration, the absence of spontaneous breathing, and the absence of central pulse.

2.2 Mobilization and transport of traumatized patients

The means of transport of patients play an important role in the specific care of these patients, transport being an integral part of the therapeutic attitude toward them.

It is also very important to know that choosing and using an inadequate means of extraction or transportation can compromise the rest of the therapeutic benefits of therapy and hence the chances of patient survival or functional recovery.

The criteria for choosing the means of transportation for these patients are as follows:

- Type of clinical situation (medical or traumatic)

- Profile and complexity of lesions

- The workspace, the ability to improvise certain types of grooves

- The quality of the access road to the destination hospital

- The need to adopt particular transport items

- The need to decide in the case of accidents with multiple victims

Particular transport positions:

- Trendelenburg—lying on an oblique plane with lower limbs higher than the head—patient in shock

- Dorsal decubitus, with perfect spine immobilization—patient with multiple trauma

All means of transport used by prehospital rescuers must have several features such as the following [1–3]:

- Easy to handle

- Light

- Not breakable

- Easy to clean

- Strong

- Having adequate dimensions at the waist of the patient

The means that can be used to transport patients are as follows:

- Stretcher

- Rigid stretcher

- Brancards

- Vacuum mattress

In HEMS transport, particular care should be provided to the hemodynamic status of patients, and a periarrest situation should be avoided because of the big difficulty of performing high-quality CPR during flight (the space for medical crew and patients is very limited in most helicopters used for medical missions).

Because of this, a systematic approach is recommended, and the crew should assess the patient carefully and deliver medical treatment for all the situations that can induce cardiorespiratory arrest during flight. To achieve this goal, we recommend using the following algorithm, utilized for primary assessment of trauma patients, which will help the medical crew to have a systematic and standardized approach [1, 2]:

- Airway

- Breathing

- Circulation

- Disabilities

- Environmental

2.3 Airway assessment and management

Ensure an open airway and protect the cervical spine.

The release and maintenance of a free airway are priorities in the treatment of any patient.

If the patient is conscious and speaks effortlessly and without overdrive sounds, the airway is probably not obstructed. If the sound is distorted or the patient makes an important effort to talk, it means a compromised airway: snoring suggests mechanical obstruction, while gurgling indicates the presence of fluid in the air (blood, secretions, and vomiting). In case of laryngeal lesions, hoarseness and/or dysphonia may occur [1–3].

The unconscious patient, with an unassured airway, may suddenly present obstruction when the base of the tongue falls into the hypopharynx. In addition, the absence of the gag reflex is an important risk for aspiration to the unconscious patient and should be a signal for the need of orotracheal intubation.

Oxygen will be administered as soon as the airway has been opened and secured by means, methods, flows, pressures, and flow adapted to the situation. In some cases, complex ventilation management is required: mechanically assisted or controlled ventilation, intratracheal aspiration, pneumothorax, adequate positioning, and stabilization of flail chest, without which simple ventilation assistance or control fails to achieve or even worsen mood [1–3].

Even in traumatized patients who spontaneously breathe, the oxygen will be administered rapidly on the face mask with a reservoir at a rate of 10–15 l/min, to obtain an FiO_2 of over 85%.

Before transporting the patient, be sure that the following conditions are fulfilled [1, 2, 5]:

- Insert an airway or endotracheal tube, if needed. Proceed to orotracheal intubation in patients with altered GCS, less than 9, but also even equal or above, when there are conditions for potential deterioration during transport, especially in case of air transport.

- Use or be prepared for suction at airway level.

- Place a gastric tube in all intubated patients and in nonintubated patients with evidence of gastric distention. Decrease by all means the risk of vomiting and aspiration.

2.4 Breathing evaluation and control

Breathing assessment addresses the following major issues: the presence of spontaneous breathing, its efficacy, the respiratory rate, the pathological types of respiration requiring correction or the immediate ventilator support, and the existence of signs suggesting the existence of these highly potential lethal lesions [1, 2, 5]:

- Obstruction of upper airways

- Tension pneumothorax

- Open pneumothorax

- Flail chest

- Massive hemothorax

Detecting these lethal lesions urgently requires appropriate management, as described below:

2.4.1 Tension pneumothorax

For tension pneumothorax, treatment can be started with needle decompression, is fast, and can be performed by most personnel on ambulance but has a limited value. The thickness of the chest wall makes decompression ineffective in a significant proportion of patients. The cannula is also prone to twisting and jamming. Any attempt to decompress with a needle should be followed by the introduction of a chest drainage tube [1, 2, 5].

Next in line is the simple thoracostomy, which is easy to perform, and it consists of the first stage of insertion of the chest drainage—a simple incision and rapid dissection in the pleural space. The insertion of the chest drain is then performed. This requires additional equipment; it takes longer to carry it out and creates a closed system that has the potential to re-tension. Also, the risk of chest drainage tubes becoming clogged by blood clots exists.

We want to emphasize that a simple pneumothorax can be transformed into a tension pneumothorax when a patient is intubated and positive pressure is ventilated before decompressing the pneumothorax with a chest drainage tube! [1, 2, 5].

2.4.2 Open pneumothorax

For initial management of an open pneumothorax, promptly close the defect with a sterile dressing large enough to overlap the wound's edges. Any improvised occlusive dressing may be used as temporary measure to enable rapid assessment to continue. Fix it with tape on only three sides to provide a flutter-valve effect. As the patient inhales, the dressing occludes the wound, preventing air from entering. During exhalation, the open end of the dressing allows air to evacuate from the pleural space, and the patient will remain with a small pneumothorax. Taping all four edges of the dressing can cause air to accumulate in the thoracic cavity, resulting in a tension pneumothorax unless a chest tube is in place. Place a chest drainage tube (not on the wound!) as soon as possible [1, 2, 5, 6].

2.4.3 Massive hemothorax

Management of massive hemothorax require the insertion of a chest drain tube, the blood from pleural space, (if pleural space is not contaminated) can be collected in a collector bag and utilize for auto-transfusion on site if necessary [1, 3].

2.4.4 Flail chest

The outcome of flail chest injury is in function of associated injuries. Isolated flail chest may be successfully managed with external stabilization, but in severe flail chest, it is recommended to use also internal stabilization measure (positive end-expiratory pressure—PEEP ventilation), until thoracic surgical intervention [1, 2, 5, 7].

If there is a suspicion that airways cannot be maintained opened or there is a lesion that causes or has potential to cause inflammation at the pharyngeal level, orotracheal intubation is indicated before the development of ventilator dysfunction.

The general indications of advanced airway management in traumatized emergency patients are as follows:

- Apnea

- GCS below 9 or above, but decreasing by more than 2 points/hour

- Severe or moderate cranial trauma, to prevent secondary brain injury

- Severe facial trauma—Le Fort II/III

- Airway burn with the development of glottis edema

- The need for hyperventilation, including neurological trauma/hyperoxygenation in severe intoxication with CO

- Grade III-IV hemorrhagic shock

- Respiratory rate greater than 35/min

- Arterial gases: PaO_2 below 70 mmHg, $PaCO_2$ above 55 mmHg

- The need for general anesthesia (including stabilization of the cervical spine, access to the surgery room, and transfer or transport to long-term investigations)

- Pulmonary aspiration risk due to gastric reflux

Before transporting patients, be sure that the following conditions are fulfilled [1, 2, 5]:

- Assess the quality of breathing and administer supplementary oxygen.

- Use mechanical ventilation when needed.

- Insert a chest tube if needed. It is mandatory for patients with pneumothorax (diagnosed or suspicioned) to have a chest drainage tube placed when they are being moved by air transport.

2.5 Circulation evaluation and fluid resuscitation

Blood volume, cardiac output, and active bleeding are major circulatory issues to consider. Active hemorrhage is one of the most important causes of preventable deaths after a trauma event, immediately after tension pneumothorax.

Cardiac output can be severely decreased because of cardiac tamponade, and this is the other important finding in circulation assessment, after trauma events [1–5].

2.5.1 Bleeding

Identifying, quickly controlling hemorrhage, and initiating fluid resuscitation are crucial steps in assessing and managing circulation.

The following are the elements that provide information over the quality of the circulation during the primary assessment:

- The level of consciousness

- The color of the skin

- Pulse (quality, frequency, and regularity)

Tachycardia and hypotension are usually signs of hypovolemia. Any clinical shock signs in a traumatized patient will be assumed and treated at first as a hypovolemic shock and may be accompanied by other forms of shock encountered in the trauma: neurogenic and obstructive shock due to suffocating pneumothorax and/or cardiac tamponade.

For the early treatment of hypovolemic shock, place 2 i.v. cannulas (at least 14 g), stable and safe, at the peripherals, and start crystalline and colloid administration if necessary.

The hemostasis of the visible and approachable bleeding sources should be performed: first by applying direct pressure on the wound followed by compressive bandage, hemostatic substances, or in extremis a tourniquet. The use of tranexamic acid in the prehospital setting improved survival when this drug is administered within 3 h of injury. The first dose is usually given over 10 min and is administered in the field; the follow-up dose of 1 g is given over 8 h [1, 2, 5, 8].

For internal hemorrhages, especially intra-abdominal, hemodynamic compensation cannot be obtained even if large volumes of solutions are administered, so the patient should be transported as quickly as possible to the trauma center for emergency surgery, assisting vital functions.

Administration of type O negative blood outside the hospital, although controversial, may be a savior measure for internal hemorrhages with the loss of over 40% of the circulating volume or where hemodynamic stabilization cannot be achieved by massive administration of crystals and colloids in 10–15 min [1–5].

2.5.2 Cardiac tamponade

Cardiac tamponade can develop slowly, allowing for a less urgent evaluation, or rapidly, requiring rapid diagnosis and treatment. The classic clinical triad of Beck, muffled heart sounds, hypotension, and distended jugulars veins, is not uniformly present with cardiac tamponade. Muffled heart sounds are difficult to assess in the noisy environment, and distended neck veins may be absent due to associated hypovolemia. When cardiac tamponade is diagnosed, emergency thoracotomy or sternotomy should be performed by a qualified surgeon as soon as possible. Administration of intravenous fluid will improve cardiac output transiently. If surgical intervention is not possible, pericardiocentesis (guided by ultrasound if possible) can be therapeutic, but it does not constitute definitive treatment for cardiac tamponade [1, 3, 5, 9].

Before transporting a patient, be sure that following conditions are fulfilled:

- Control external bleeding and when a tourniquet is used note on a label the time of placement.

- Establish two large-caliber intravenous lines and begin crystalloid solution infusion.

- Restore blood volume losses using crystalloid fluid and blood and continue replacement during transfer.

- Insert a urinary catheter to monitor urine output.

- Monitor the patient's cardiac rhythm and rate.

2.6 Disability (neurologic evaluation)

A rapid neurologic evaluation will establish the patient's level of consciousness by using Glasgow Coma Score (GCS), will assess pupillary size and reaction to light, identifies the presence of lateralizing signs, and should asses the presence of spinal cord injury and the level of the injury, if it is present.

The control of the spine and especially of the cervical spine is initiated with the primary evaluation of the vital functions, respectively with the opening of the airways, from the first contact with the patient [1, 3, 5].

This element is extremely important, as it is known that amielic lesions of the cervical spine can easily transform into mielic lesions by inappropriate maneuvers or mielic lesions may worsen (including hypoxia, edema, or hypovolemia) leading to medullary sections. Patients who will benefit from cervical column immobilization are those [1, 3, 5]:

- who are involved in road traffic accidents;

- who are involved in a fall from height;

- who require extrication measure (usually in car accidents);

- who are traumatized with obvious injuries to the throat from striking, shooting, or stabbing;

- whose symptomatology indicates a cervical spine injury (localized pain in the spine, functional impotence, limb paresthesia or anesthesia, priapism, bulbocavernosus reflex, anal reflex, upper abdominal skin reflexes, etc.);

- who are in a mentally altered status, when the mechanism of production of the traumatic event cannot be specified.

In all these patients, the methods of protection and then immobilization of the cervical spine, as well as the special methods of extraction, mobilization, and transportation of traumatized patients, will be applied as follows [1, 3, 5]:

- Manually protecting the cervical spine by keeping the head, neck, and trunk in the axle. Manual control of the cervical spine will be maintained throughout the orotracheal intubation, which, in case of suspected cervical lesion, is a difficult maneuver, requiring Sellick maneuver.

- The stiff neck will be placed immediately after the manual fitting of the head. The stiff neck is used to protect the column against flexion-extension movements, less than the lateral and almost none of the rotation, which is why the manual protection should be maintained even after the stiff neck is placed.

- The rigid column strap with head side stabilizers and the front and lumbar fastening bands is used to achieve complete immobilization of the spine after patient evaluation and airways management have been performed and the patient is ready for extraction and transport.

- The vacuum mattress is an alternative to the rigid stretcher, especially for the patient with multiple trauma who also presents the instability of the pelvic area.

Before transporting a patient, be sure that the following conditions are fulfilled [1, 3, 5]:

- Secure airway and assist breathing in unconscious patients.

- Administer mannitol or hypertonic saline, if needed.

- Restrict spinal motion in patients who have or are suspected of having spine injuries.

2.7 Exposure and environmental control

During the primary assessment, undress the patient and it is advisable to cut off clothes to facilitate a thorough examination and assessment without producing or aggravating injuries. Watch out for hypothermia; this situation can appear very fast in a trauma patient [1, 3].

After completing the assessment, cover the patient with warm blankets or an external warming device to prevent developing hypothermia. Because hypothermia is a potentially lethal complication in case of trauma patients, take all the measures necessary to prevent the loss of body heat and restore body temperature to normal.

Also, during this final step of primary assessment, if it is possible, it is recommended to find the circumstances that produce the traumatic event (trauma cinematics). According to this finding, it is possible to presume that the most probable injury occurred after the traumatic event.

2.8 Final general aspects

The number of patients who developed cardiac arrest caused by trauma or accidental injury is increasing, and the number of potentially preventable prehospital deaths produced in traumatic circumstances seems to remain statistically high, despite major advances achieved in trauma care.

Bystanders witness the event in most of the cases, but while making the call for medical assistance, first aid intervention of any kind is infrequent. It is clear that there exists a time following injury when the bystander has an opportunity to provide first aid before the arrival of the EMS, which could potentially improve outcomes. The window of instructions provided by the dispatch to the witness could improve the surviving rate and output of the trauma patient (e.g., recommendation to move a trauma patient, if permitted, and how to move him correctly, and recommendation of how to correctly open and maintain a clear airway). Lay personnel first aid measure including simple airway management and ventilation support during this window of time without any therapeutic measures could significantly improve survival.

The prehospital care community needs to agree to a consensus on how to define and determine the preventability of death in the prehospital phase and to enable detailed study of each of the prehospital phases in order to improve current practice [9, 10].

It is described in literature that implementation of a physician-staffed helicopter was associated with significantly reduced delay for arrival at the level I trauma center of severely injured trauma patients. The proportion of secondary transfer and 30-day mortality were also significantly reduced [11, 12].

The preponderance of recent and previous scientific evidence supports an argument that the HEMS transport is associated with significant benefit for some injured patients. The primary challenges at this moment include the determination of which patients benefit and to find of which aspects of the HEMS are responsible for any salutary effects of its utilization [13]. A top-level type of prehospital care had significantly more chances to resuscitate blunt trauma victims found in CA as compared with a simpler level [14].

Also, there are evidence of an association between helicopter transport mode and increased survival in blunt trauma patients [15].

Anyway, the role and structure of HEMS in the modern trauma service are a debate that is likely to continue. Prehospital care design should be specific to critical incident frequency, geographical particularity of hospital facilities, and travel times within each trauma network. It is also important to consider the benefits, expertise, and capabilities of the emergency medical team separately from the transport method.

An effective HEMS intervention will ultimately depend on effective operating procedures and tasking protocols, clinical governance, and auditing of the HEMS activity. Future work in this area should also examine the costs and safety of HEMS, since multiple contextual determinants must be considered when evaluating the effects of HEMS for adults with major trauma [16–18].

3. Conclusions

A systematic approach following a standardized protocol is recommended to be applied in case of trauma patients.

The actual recommendation is to asses quickly, at the first contact, the patient (primary assessment), delivering at the same time the necessary treatment for life-threatening situations. The approach algorithm for this primary assessment is described as ABCDE approach (Airway, Breathing, Circulation, Disabilities, and Exposure).

All the life-threatening injuries should be recognized during primary assessment and the required treatment should be applied as soon as possible, without any delay.

This step will be followed by a secondary assessment, this time a complete clinical examination, concomitant with continuously monitoring vital function, and frequent reassessment.

Obtaining intravenous access, beginning fluid resuscitation, and applying oxygen from the first moments could be lifesaving measures, and this simple procedure creates time for more complex and definitive procedures.

Providing advanced airway management is one of the top priorities of trauma care. Management of difficult airway requires technical expertise, but also, the decision of when and how to approach airway is equally important, which are the determinants of outcome. Again, we want to emphasize that a pneumothorax will be transformed into a tension pneumothorax, which can be followed by cardiac arrest, if a patient is orotracheally intubated and mechanically ventilated before decompressing the pneumothorax with a chest drainage tube.

Another essential thing to do during patient transfer is prehospital information delivery by radio or phone to the receiving hospital. This report should include the cause and the circumstances of the accident, the patient's condition upon arrival of the emergency physician on scene, medical measures provided at the site of the accident and during transport, prior diseases and any history of patient if available, and complications.

The role and structure of HEMS in the modern trauma service are still in a debate that probably will continue. Prehospital care needs to be specific to critical incident frequency, geographical situation of hospital facilities, and travel times necessary to reach the nearest trauma center. Also, it is very important to consider the benefits and capabilities of the emergency medical team separately from the transport method.

An effective transport care (using ground transport or helicopter) will ultimately depend on effective operating procedures and trauma protocols, clinical local guides, and auditing of the crew's (ambulance or helicopter) EMS activity.

Conflict of interest

The authors declare no conflict of interest.

Author details

Tudor Ovidiu Popa[1,2]*, Diana Carmen Cimpoesu[1,2] and Paul Lucian Nedelea[1,2]

1 University of Medicine and Pharmacy Grigore T. Popa, Iasi, Romania

2 Emergency Department, Emergency County Hospital Sf. Spiridon, Iasi, Romania

*Address all correspondence to: ovidiupopa8@gmail.com

References

[1] Cimpoesu D, Popa O, Petris A, et al. Current Protocols and Guidelines in Emergency Medicine. Iasi: UMF "Gr. T. Popa" Publishing House; 2011

[2] Truhlář A, Deakin CD, Soar J, et al. European Resuscitation Council Guidelines for Resuscitation 2015: Section 4. Cardiac arrest in special circumstances. Resuscitation. 2015;**95**:148-201. DOI: 10.1016/j.resuscitation.2015.07.017

[3] Cameron P, Knapp BJ. Trauma in adults. In: Tintinalli JE, editor. Tintinalli's Emergency Medicine: A Comprehensive Study Guide. 8th ed. New York: McGraw-Hill Publishing House; 2016. ISBN: 007179476X

[4] Bloom BA, Gibbons RC. Focused Assessment with Sonography for Trauma (FAST). Treasure Island, FL: StatPearls Publishing; 2019. Available from: https://www.ncbi.nlm.nih.gov/books/NBK470479/

[5] Stewart RM, editor. Advanced Trauma Life Support. 10th ed. Chicago: American College of Surgeons; 2018. ISBN 78-0-9968262-3-5

[6] Roberts D, Leigh-Smith S, Faris P, et al. Clinical presentation of patients with tension pneumothorax: A systematic review. Annals of Surgery. 2015;**261**(6):1068-1078. DOI: 10.1097/SLA.0000000000001073

[7] Simon B, Ebert J, Bokhari F, et al. Management of pulmonary contusion and flail chest: An Eastern Association for the Surgery of Trauma practice management guideline. Journal of Trauma and Acute Care Surgery. 2012;**73**(5):S351-S361. DOI: 10.1097/TA.0b013e31827019fd

[8] CRASH-2 collaborators, Roberts I, Shakur H, et al. The importance of early treatment with tranexamic acid in bleeding trauma patients: An exploratory analysis of the CRASH-2 randomized controlled trial. Lancet. 2011;**377**(9771):1096-1101. DOI: 10.1016/S0140-6736(11)60278-X

[9] Hunt PA, Greaves I, Owens WA. Emergency thoracotomy in thoracic trauma—A review. Injury. 2006;**37**(1):1-19. DOI: 10.1016/j.injury.2005.02.014

[10] Oliver GJ et al. Are prehospital deaths from trauma and accidental injury preventable? A direct historical comparison to assess what has changed in two decades. Injury;**48**(5):978-984. DOI: 10.1016/j.injury.2017.01.039

[11] Hesselfeldt R, Steinmetz J, et al. Impact of a physician-staffed helicopter on a regional trauma system: A prospective, controlled, observational study. Acta Anaesthesiologica Scandinavica. 2013;**57**:660-668. DOI: 10.1111/aas.12052

[12] Shepherd MV, Trethewy CE, et al. Helicopter use in rural trauma. Emergency Medicine Australasia. 2008;**20**(6):494-499. DOI: 10.1111/j.1742-6723.2008.01135.x

[13] Thomas S, Biddinger P, et al. Helicopter trauma transport: An overview of recent outcomes and triage literature. Current Opinion in Anaesthesiology. 2003;**16**(2):153-158

[14] Di BS, Sanson G, Nardi G, et al. Hems vs. Ground-Bls care in traumatic cardiac arrest. Prehospital Emergency Care. 2005;**9**(1):79-84. DOI: 10.1080/10903120590891886

[15] Thomas SH, Harrison T, et al. Helicopter transport and blunt trauma mortality: A multicenter trial. The Journal of Trauma: Injury, Infection, and Critical Care. 2002;**52**(1):136-145

[16] Butler DP, Anwar I, Willett K. Is it the H or the EMS in HEMS that has an impact on trauma patient mortality? A systematic review of the evidence. Emergency Medicine Journal. 2010;**27**:692-701. DOI: 10.1136/emj.2009.087486

[17] Galvagno SM Jr, Sikorski R, Hirshon JM, Floccare D, Stephens C, Beecher D, et al. Helicopter emergency medical services for adults with major trauma. Cochrane Database of Systematic Reviews. 2015;(12). Article ID: CD009228. DOI: 10.1002/14651858. CD009228.pub3

[18] Frink M, Probst C, Hildebrand F, et al. The influence of transportation mode on mortality in polytraumatized patients. An analysis based on the German Trauma Registry. Der Unfallchirurg. 2007;**110**(4):334-340. DOI: 10.1007/s00113-006-1222-2

Section 2

Hospital Management of Trauma

Chapter 4

Treatment Toxicity: Radiation

Thomas J. FitzGerald, Maryann Bishop-Jodoin, Fran Laurie,
Matthew Iandoli, Ameer Elaimy, James Shen, Peter Lee,
Alexander Lukez, Lakshmi Shanmugham, Beth Herrick,
Jon Glanzman and David Goff

Abstract

Radiation exposures, both intentional and unintentional, have influence on normal tissue function. Short-term and long-term injuries can occur to all cell systems of both limited and rapid self-renewal potential. Radiation effects can last a lifetime for a patient and can produce complications for all organs and systems. Often invisible at the time of exposure, the fingerprints for cell damage can appear at any timepoint after. Health-care providers will need comprehensive knowledge and understanding of the acute and late effects of radiation exposure and how these interrelate with immediate and long-term care.

Keywords: radiation exposure, cell damage, toxicity, radiation dose/volume

1. Introduction

Radiation exposure can occur during diagnosis and primary treatment of a cancer or during a nuclear incident. These exposures increase our need to educate health-care providers and first responders on assessing and managing patients [1–8]. Although effects on tissue may not be meaningful from a clinical perspective during an evaluation for healthcare, identification of radiation exposure from a dose and volume perspective is an important piece in the patient's past medical history. Invisible fingerprints relevant to medical situations can declare themselves decades after exposure in spite of careful periodic evaluation. The dose and volume of the intentional exposure is usually well documented in the radiation therapy treatment record. Shadow parallel radiation records that are not entered into electronic health system records may not be available at the time of a related health-care evaluation, and important clinical information may be too brief or inadequate. Many current electronic medical records (EMR) do not have a module for radiation oncology. Data acquisition and management of radiation oncology are conducted with proprietary software systems and are not directly included in the modern electronic record. Interfaces can be built to move small portions of records to the EMR; however these are not reliable modes of data transfer and, if transferred, often cannot be easily retrieved when needed in the acute care setting. Unintentional exposure including exposure from diagnostic imaging is more challenging to document as it is provider-dependent and limited reliable information is documented during a radiology procedure. Radiation dose exposure is estimated using distance and duration models from the primary source as victims, unlike health-care providers, are frequently unmonitored [1–4, 6, 8]. While these estimation models may be useful, accuracy can be compromised, particularly in calculating the integral or total body dose as there are often multiple sources of radiation at the time of the unintended exposure along with thermal injury. With the increasing rate of cancer survivors and the transition of pediatric patients to adult care systems, there is a multilevel knowledge gap of the toxicities caused by radiation exposure and how the acute and late effects relate to patient care.

2. Radiation toxicity

2.1 Normal tissue damage

We arbitrarily categorize radiation injury into phases: acute injury (3 months from exposure), subacute (from 3 to 24 months from exposure), and late or chronic (>24 months from exposure). There is considerable overlap in these definitions, and acute injury can be less and non-predictive of chronic injury [1–4]. Acute intentional injuries, both expected and unanticipated, related to radiation therapy management of cancer are best managed by the responsible treating physicians during radiation treatment. These professionals are cognizant of the intended target and normal tissues in the treatment field. Their knowledge of radiation treatment's impact on normal tissue is coupled with established and less well-established toxicities with various applications of chemotherapy and targeted therapy. Unintentional radiation exposure requires additional support and evaluation by emergency services working together with radiation safety experts, who are trained in managing radiation effects and assessing the dose received by the victims using models of time and distance from the epicenter of the event. This also includes evaluating the risk to caregivers of the victim if radioactive particles/elements remain on or in the victim. The acute phase of injury can affect many cell systems. This includes toxicity to limited and rapid self-renewal potential tissues such as the central nervous system, bone marrow, skin, and mucosal surfaces lining the head/neck and gastrointestinal system. Death can occur soon after exposure if it is not recognized in a timely manner and appropriate support is not provided. Although injury to reticulum systems is less common from radiation exposure due to limited self-renewal of these cell systems, injury to these systems including thermal injury eliminate the scaffolding needed for structural repair of cell systems with rapid self-renewal potential as disorderly repair can severely limit cell function.

From an individual cellular perspective, radiation therapy has direct impact on intracellular molecules and can cause both single-strand and double-strand DNA breaks which are repaired through multiple mechanisms. Because water is an important intracellular compound, oxygen compounds including free radical formation creates injury to cells through ionization from radiation exposure. These processes are important for cells and groups of cells near each other. The significance of the injury is directly related to the volume of tissue injured from the exposure as well as the degree of injury to support cells (stroma) that often have a more limited self-renewal capacity. If stroma is significantly damaged, cells with rapid self-renewal potential will not have a support architecture to reorganize and maintain function. The seriousness of acute and late injury is also proportional to the dose and volume of tissue exposed. Late injury is manifested by accelerated fibrosis coupled with limited blood vessel proliferation. The mechanism of late injury is multifactorial in origin including damage to rapid and limited self-renewal potential tissues, blood vessels, and intrinsic repair capacity of the cell system injured mitigated by mechanisms that accelerate fibrosis including TGF beta [9].

Radiation exposure symptoms differ with the severity of the exposure. At very high single-fraction total body doses (>10 Gy (Gray)), near-immediate death will occur through cerebrovascular syndrome despite medical care. The syndrome is due to profound edema within the brain and meninges associated with collapse of all neuromuscular processes due to swelling and herniation of the brain through the foramen magnum. At total body doses of 5–12 Gy, death without support will occur within a few weeks as a result of profound fluid loss and diarrhea due to denudation and destruction of the gastrointestinal system. This can affect both stem cells and cause secondary injury to subdermal structures deforming the architecture of the bowel inhibiting absorption and promoting fluid loss. Patient survival is directly correlated with gastrointestinal (fluid/nutrition) and bone marrow (blood/blood product) support during this phase after exposure. A single total body dose of 10 Gy will eradicate a large segment of the stem cells within the gastrointestinal crypts. Although this dose does not directly affect differentiated adult cells, the exposure eliminates the stem cell self-renewal potential; therefore, the gastrointestinal tract mucosal surface becomes denuded, and the reticulum architecture supporting cell organization can be damaged. As a result, with no barrier for fluid and blood loss, clinical deterioration will occur often within days. At total body exposure doses of 2–5 Gy, death occurs from destruction to the hematopoietic system with primary damage to both stem cells and cells of established lineation. Cells cannot sustain self-renewal, and clinical deterioration can occur with primary marrow failure and secondary infection. Lymphocytes may die an intermitotic death; thus the degree of lymphopenia can provide indirect assessment of dose from exposure [1, 5–8].

During exposure, symptoms consistent with a radiation syndrome will be developed by the victim and can be seen as early as 15 minutes from the initial exposure [1, 6, 8]. Symptom severity is proportional to dose. At higher doses, victims can experience severe gastrointestinal fluid loss, secondary fever from exposure to homeopathic pathogens, and hypotension due to fluid loss suggesting significant toxicity. Often identified at lower dose exposure, the prodromal phase is followed by a latent interval during which the person may look and feel clinically well for days to weeks. After this gastrointestinal and hematopoietic damage may become visible and require intervention to prevent further acute clinical deterioration [1, 5–8].

If the total body exposure is <4–5 Gy, most experts currently recommend no immediate intervention other than symptomatic treatment with fluids and blood support. This would include periodic hydration and antiemetic therapy for nausea and vomiting. As needed, infection can be treated with antibiotics. Death associated with the hematopoietic syndrome becomes a real concern for exposure >5 Gy. Barrier nursing intervention and appropriate blood product support may improve survival. Experience from recent nuclear events suggest that efforts to limit bleeding, infection, and physical trauma during the blood count nadir may improve the LD 50/30 (50% survival at 30 days) to and possibly beyond 7 Gy.

Dermal surfaces can receive much higher doses than internal organs, particularly if the exposure is related to particles. Dermal injuries can be primitive dose biomarkers with epilation/erythema at 3–6 Gy and wet desquamation, bullae, ulceration, and necrosis visible at increased doses [1, 10]. However, if the exposure is a contaminate of radioactive particle and photon exposure, dermal dose may not be an accurate assessment of total body dose. Dermal injuries can be life-threatening due to concurrent infection. Injuries should be managed with the same care offered to burn victims with care taken to monitor health-care staff in case there are residual particles which can transmit unintentional dose to health-care providers. Residual exposure can be identified with careful monitoring with dosimeters as done in brachytherapy treatments for health-care providers.

An accurate assessment of dose is very important during the triage and care of victims with unintended exposure. Health-care workers are often monitored with dosimeters; however, the public will not have access to these tools. Therefore, radiation exposure and dose assessment experts are important early in the evaluation including analysis of the population at risk. As radiation dose increases, the time to emesis decreases, and rapid onset of nausea and vomiting suggests higher exposure. As indicated, a decline in lymphocyte count or abnormal lymphocyte cytogenetics can be an indirect estimate of dose within 1–2 days of exposure. [1, 6–8, 11]. The Radiation Emergency Assistance Center for the United States (US) Department of Energy is operated by Oak Ridge Institute for Science and Education. Medical and radiation safety support is available through a 24-hour consultation service. Resources include radiation dose assessment in laboratory facilities and computation of dose from radionucleotide expertise. The 24-hour emergency telephone number is 865.576.3131, and the website is https://orise.orau.gov/reacts/resources/index.html.

Recognized as an important clinical endeavor since nuclear weapons have been developed, there is keen interest in finding the chemical compounds that can protect normal tissues against radiation injury. Radiation protectors are compounds applied or administered prior to exposure or in selected circumstances soon thereafter, to limit the impact and subsequent damage from exposure upon normal tissue. Compounds that can influence and promote the health of normal tissue after exposure are referred to as radiation mitigators. These therapeutic compounds are applied once the injury has occurred. Sulfhydryl compounds (SHs) have been shown to be effective radioprotectors. The simplest of these compounds, cysteine, contains a natural amino acid [11, 12]. The mechanism is thought to be related to the augmentation of amino acids in generating repair proteins at a higher level. Once the compound becomes intracellular, it loses the phosphate group and is thought to also serve as a free radical scavenger limiting intracellular damage.

Amifostine (ethyol) has been used to prevent xerostomia in patients receiving radiation therapy for head and neck cancer [13]. Several clinical trials have used amifostine to evaluate the effectiveness in protecting multiple mucosal surfaces as well as protecting pulmonary injury in patients undergoing total body irradiation therapy as part of bone marrow transplant [13]. Amifostine was associated with improvement in patient assessment of mouth dryness and swallowing in a trial managed by the National Clinical Trial Network [13, 14]. The intrinsic fear of applying radiation protectors and mitigators in cancer therapy is the possible simultaneous tumor protective effect of these compounds in situ potentially limiting the usefulness of the compounds. In this trial, it is important to note there was no difference in tumor control between patients receiving amifostine and patients receiving placebo. Nitroxides have been identified by Citrin and colleagues [11] as radioprotection agents in clinical development. Stable nitroxide free radicals and their specific electron reduction products, hydroxylamines, protect cells when exposed to oxidative stress. Accordingly, similar compounds are under review and evaluation. Antioxidants, such as alpha-tocopherol and beta-carotene, are under review for clinical application but to date have not been shown to be of clinical benefit [15, 16]. Investigators explored using gene therapy vectors with superoxide dismutase (SOD) to improve the intracellular component of SOD. The purpose is to limit damage caused by superoxide radicals. Investigators have demonstrated improved normal tissue tolerance to multiple organs including the esophagus with this approach [17, 18]. Captopril is a sulfhydryl containing analog of proline and inhibits angiotensin-converting enzyme and limits vasoconstriction. In animal models, it has been shown to benefit renal and pulmonary function with total body irradiation by limiting endothelial dysfunction, fluid exudation, and the subsequent development of pulmonary fibrosis. It also appeared to improve recovery of hematoprogenitor cells [19–21]. ON 01210 (chlorobenzylsulfone derivative) is a small molecule kinase inhibitor which potentiates recovery of peripheral blood elements when administered before radiation. This may be of benefit to the general public and first responders in an unanticipated event if received early postexposure [22]. Animal models have shown a positive repopulation effect of gastrointestinal stem cells with R-spondin 1, a 263 amino acid protein [23]. CBLB502 is an agent that binds to toll-like receptor 5 (TLR5) activating NF-kB signal pathways. It is derived from the flagellin protein of *Salmonella* bacteria. It promotes recovery and regeneration of multiple organ system stem cells after TBI therapy including GI, oral mucosa, skin, and bone marrow progenitors. IL-6 and other bone marrow-associated colony-stimulating factors likewise appear to work in parallel with this compound. The compound has a potential role as both a protectant and a mitigator [24]. Gamma-tocotrienol is an isomer of vitamin E and supports survival in animal models during total body irradiation in part by promoting bone marrow colony-stimulating factors and IL-6. It also may play a role in upregulating anti-apoptotic gene expression after radiation [25, 26].

The role of mitigators is to limit injury from radiation exposure prior to the clinical manifestations of acute and late toxicities of the exposure and treatment. These compounds are generally thought to influence metabolic events occurring after exposure and limit radiation-associated damage. To date, cytokines and growth factors directed to stimulate stem cell proliferation are the most common tools used for this purpose. In clinical practice, these are commonly used to balance the inhibition of stem cell growth induced by chemotherapy and radiation to the hematopoietic, dermal, and gastrointestinal systems. These include granulocyte colony-stimulating factor (G-CSF) and keratinocyte growth factor (KGF) [27]. The factors contribute to many aspects of cell recovery. KGF has positive influence in the recovery of mucosal surfaces during the acute phase of toxicity as well as limits the late effects of radiotherapy, including xerostomia [11]. This is thought to potentially be of benefit to patients undergoing primary management for head and neck tumors. Mitigators of late toxicity are largely directed to limit fibrosis, which is thought to be a primary factor in late pulmonary injury and other tissues of more limited self-renewal potential [11, 15–18, 28–32]. Transforming growth factor beta (TGF-B) is the primary target to limit fibrosis [33–35]. Several compounds in development prevent late effects to either directly or indirectly target the TGF-B signaling pathway [33–35]. Tumor protection remains a concern when evaluating treatments associated with this parallel pathway for patients being treated for a malignancy, identical to compounds associated with radiation protection. There has been increasing interest in the use of stem cell therapy to repair both acute and chronic injuries. Mesenchymal stem cells modified with extracellular superoxide dismutase have been shown to improve survival of irradiated mice [36]. There is evidence these progenitors have a pleuripotent role and can be called upon by organ systems for differentiation along multiple pathways. Bone marrow stromal cells and myeloid progenitors are also under evaluation to mitigate radiation response. The survival benefit in mice with infusion of myeloid progenitors could be seen days after exposure [37–40]. The role of these infusional therapies in this circumstance remains to be optimally defined. The role of transplant and stem cell infusion during the Chernobyl crisis was uncertain; however these techniques have improved and remain to be optimized in similar situations moving forward.

Neutrophil inhibition has the potential of limiting the severity of response to injury, and this has been evaluated in a series of experiments determining the potential role of these strategic compounds applied after radiation exposure. Experiments evaluated interleukin-1 alpha (IL-1α) as a mitigator of dermal damage after radiation exposure. Interleukin-1 (IL-1) inhibits neutrophil infiltration into the initial inflammatory response to injury. Assuming the initial inflammatory phase can be titrated, short-term and long-term injuries could be influenced. Knockout mice deficient in IL-1α or the IL-1 receptor demonstrated both decreased dermal injury and more rapid healing after superficial radiation exposure with both electrons and a strontium applicator. This demonstrated the potential importance of this cytokine in generating and ameliorating radiation-associated skin damage associated with neutrophil inhibition. In a separate group of experiments, investigators demonstrated that hyperspectral optical imaging (HSI) can reveal acute and late oxygenation and perfusion changes in dermal tissue with changes occurring as early as 12 hours after radiation exposure [41, 42]. Imaging changes in oxygenation and perfusion were seen within 12 hours of exposure and predated clinical visible skin change by 14 days [42]. Data sets from this group as part of an approved Institutional Review Board clinical trial for breast cancer patients receiving radiation therapy have shown that changes in imaging correlate well with radiation dose and dose asymmetry in the treated volume. Areas of increased dose associated with patient topography, and chest wall separation demonstrated changes consistent with increased dose and daily fractionation.

In response to the need of developing compounds for radioprotection and mitigation, the Radiation Research Program of the National Cancer Institute in collaboration with the Small Business Innovation Research program has funded a series of contracts since 2010 to support the development of radiomodulators. To date, five of the funded applications have successfully transitioned to phase II funding. Eight clinical trials have been developed to establish safety and efficacy. Two drugs on trial are under evaluation as radioprotectors, and two are also being evaluated for anticancer properties. The sites of interest being studied include CNS injury, mucositis, proctitis/enteritis, bone marrow failure, and lung injury [43].

3. Conclusions

Researchers are developing a targeted pharmacologic response to protect and mitigate issues surrounding intentional and unintentional radiation exposure. A knowledge of normal tissue response to radiation injury will be important for all health-care providers moving forward. Radiation therapy patients, accident victims, and first responders will benefit from the growing body of knowledge.

Conflict of interest

The authors have no conflict of interest.

Author details

Thomas J. FitzGerald[1*], Maryann Bishop-Jodoin[2], Fran Laurie[2],
Matthew Iandoli[2], Ameer Elaimy[3], James Shen[3], Peter Lee[3], Alexander Lukez[3],
Lakshmi Shanmugham[4], Beth Herrick[5], Jon Glanzman[6] and David Goff[7]

1 Department of Radiation Oncology, University of Massachusetts Medical School,
UMass Memorial Managed Care Network, Worcester, MA, USA

2 Department of Radiation Oncology, University of Massachusetts Medical School,
Worcester, MA, USA

3 University of Massachusetts Medical School, Worcester, MA, USA

4 Department of Radiation Oncology, University of Massachusetts Medical School,
UMassMemorial Managed Care Network, Fitchburg, MA, USA

5 Department of Radiation Oncology, University of Massachusetts Medical School,
UMassMemorial Managed Care Network, Brighton, MA, USA

6 Department of Radiation Oncology, University of Massachusetts Medical School,
UMassMemorial Managed Care Network, Foxborough, MA, USA

7 Department of Radiation Oncology, University of Massachusetts Medical School,
UMassMemorial Managed Care Network, Methuen, MA, USA

*Address all correspondence to: tj.fitzgerald@umassmemorial.org;
thomas.fitzGerald@umassmed.edu

IntechOpen

References

[1] Hall EJ, Giaccia AJ. Radiobiology for the Radiologist. 7th ed. Philadelphia: Lippincott Williams and Wilkins; 2012. p. 576

[2] Miller DL, Balter S, Cole PE, Lu HT, Berenstein A, Albert R, et al. Radiation doses in interventional radiology procedures: The RAD-IR study: Part II: Skin dose. Journal of Vascular and Interventional Radiology. 2003;14:977-990

[3] Miller DL, Balter S, Wagner LK, Cardella J, Clark TW, Neithamer CD Jr, et al. Quality improvement guidelines for recording patient radiation dose in the medical record. Journal of Vascular and Interventional Radiology. 2004;15:423-429

[4] Shope TB. Radiation-induced skin injuries from fluoroscopy. RadioGraphics. 1996;16:1195-1199

[5] Donnelly EH, Nemhauser JB, Smith JM, Kazzi ZN, Farfan EB, Chang AS, et al. Acute radiation syndrome: Assessment and management. Southern Medical Journal. 2010;103:541-546. DOI: 10.1097/SMJ.0b013e3181ddd571

[6] Turai I, Veress K. Radiation accidents: Occurrence, types, consequences, medical management, and lessons learned. Central European Journal of Occupational and Environmental Medicine. 2001;7:3-14

[7] Baranov A, Gale RP, Guskova A, Piatkin E, Selidovkin G, Muravyova L, et al. Bone marrow transplantation after the Chernobyl nuclear accident. The New England Journal of Medicine. 1989;321:205-212. DOI: 10.1056/NEJM198907273210401

[8] Contributors W. Acute Radiation Syndrome Wikipedia, The Free Encyclopedia [Internet]. 2014. Available from: http://en.wikipedia. org/w/index.php?title=Acute_radiation_syndrome&oldid=608982279 [Accessed: April 1, 2019]

[9] Williams JP, McBride WH. After the bomb drops: A new look at radiation-induced multiple organ dysfunction syndrome (MODS). International Journal of Radiation Biology. 2011;87:851-868. DOI: 10.3109/09553002.2011.560996

[10] Fitzgerald TJ, Jodoin MB, Tillman G, Aronowitz J, Pieters R, Balducci S, et al. Radiation therapy toxicity to the skin. Dermatologic Clinics. 2008;26:161-172

[11] Citrin D, Cotrim AP, Hyodo F, Baum BJ, Krishna MC, Mitchell JB. Radioprotectors and mitigators of radiation-induced normal tissue injury. The Oncologist. 2010;15:360-371. DOI: 10.1634/theoncologist.2009-S104

[12] Patt HM, Tyree EB, Straube RL, Smith DE. Cysteine protection against x irradiation. Science. 1949;110:213-214

[13] Brizel D, Overgaard J. Does amifostine have a role in chemoradiation treatment? The Lancet Oncology. 2003;4:378-381

[14] Brizel DM, Wasserman TH, Henke M, Strnad V, Rudat V, Monnier A, et al. Phase III randomized trial of amifostine as a radioprotector in head and neck cancer. Journal of Clinical Oncology. 2000;18:3339-3345

[15] Chitra S, Shyamala Devi CS. Effects of radiation and alpha-tocopherol on saliva flow rate, amylase activity, total protein and electrolyte levels in oral cavity cancer. Indian Journal of Dental Research. 2008;19:213-218

[16] Bentzen SM. Preventing or reducing late side effects of radiation therapy: Radiobiology meets molecular pathology. Nature Reviews. Cancer. 2006;6:702-713

[17] Epperly MW, Bray JA, Krager S, Berry LM, Gooding W, Engelhardt JF, et al. Intratracheal injection of adenovirus containing the human MnSOD transgene protects athymic nude mice from irradiation-induced organizing alveolitis. International Journal of Radiation Oncology, Biology, Physics. 1999;**43**:169-181

[18] Epperly MW, Defilippi S, Sikora C, Gretton J, Kalend A, Greenberger JS. Intratracheal injection of manganese superoxide dismutase (MnSOD) plasmid/liposomes protects normal lung but not orthotopic tumors from irradiation. Gene Therapy. 2000;**7**:1011-1018

[19] Moulder JE, Cohen EP, Fish BL. Captopril and losartan for mitigation of renal injury caused by single-dose total-body irradiation. Radiation Research. 2011;**175**:29-36. DOI: 10.1667/RR2400.1

[20] Ghosh SN, Zhang R, Fish BL, Semenenko VA, Li XA, Moulder JE, et al. Renin-angiotensin system suppression mitigates experimental radiation pneumonitis. International Journal of Radiation Oncology, Biology, Physics. 2009;**75**:1528-1536. DOI: 10.1016/j.ijrobp.2009.07.1743

[21] Chisi JE, Briscoe CV, Ezan E, Genet R, Riches AC, Wdzieczak-Bakala J. Captopril inhibits in vitro and in vivo the proliferation of primitive haematopoietic cells induced into cell cycle by cytotoxic drug administration or irradiation but has no effect on myeloid leukaemia cell proliferation. British Journal of Haematology. 2000;**109**:563-570

[22] Suman S, Datta K, Doiron K, Ren C, Kumar R, Taft DR, et al. Radioprotective effects of ON 01210. Na upon oral administration. Journal of Radiation Research. 2012;**53**:368-376

[23] Bhanja P, Saha S, Kabarriti R, Liu L, Roy-Chowdhury N, Roy-Chowdhury J, et al. Protective role of R-spondin1, an intestinal stem cell growth factor, against radiation-induced gastrointestinal syndrome in mice. PLoS One. 2009;**4**:e8014. DOI: 10.1371/journal.pone.0008014

[24] Vijay-Kumar M, Aitken JD, Sanders CJ, Frias A, Sloane VM, Xu J, et al. Flagellin treatment protects against chemicals, bacteria, viruses, and radiation. Journal of Immunology. 2008;**180**:8280-8285

[25] Suman S, Datta K, Chakraborty K, Kulkarni SS, Doiron K, Fornace AJ Jr, et al. Gamma tocotrienol, a potent radioprotector, preferentially upregulates expression of anti-apoptotic genes to promote intestinal cell survival. Food and Chemical Toxicology. 2013;**60**:488-496. DOI: 10.1016/j.fct.2013.08.011

[26] Kulkarni S, Ghosh SP, Satyamitra M, Mog S, Hieber K, Romanyukha L, et al. Gamma-tocotrienol protects hematopoietic stem and progenitor cells in mice after total-body irradiation. Radiation Research. 2010;**173**:738-747. DOI: 10.1667/RR1824.1

[27] Farrell CL, Rex KL, Kaufman SA, Dipalma CR, Chen JN, Scully S, et al. Effects of keratinocyte growth factor in the squamous epithelium of the upper aerodigestive tract of normal and irradiated mice. International Journal of Radiation Biology. 1999;**75**:609-620

[28] Soule BP, Hyodo F, Matsumoto K, Simone NL, Cook JA, Krishna MC, et al. Therapeutic and clinical applications of nitroxide compounds. Antioxidants & Redox Signaling. 2007;**9**:1731-1743

[29] Hyodo F, Matsumoto K, Matsumoto A, Mitchell JB, Krishna MC. Probing the intracellular redox status of tumors with magnetic resonance imaging and redox-sensitive contrast agents. Cancer Research. 2006;**66**:9921-9928

[30] Guo H, Seixas-Silva JA Jr, Epperly MW, Gretton JE, Shin DM, Bar-Sagi D, et al. Prevention of radiation-induced oral cavity mucositis by plasmid/liposome delivery of the human manganese superoxide dismutase (SOD_2) transgene. Radiation Research. 2003;**159**:361-370

[31] Stickle RL, Epperly MW, Klein E, Bray JA, Greenberger JS. Prevention of irradiation-induced esophagitis by plasmid/liposome delivery of the human manganese superoxide dismutase transgene. Radiation Oncology Investigations. 1999;7:204-217

[32] Burdelya LG, Krivokrysenko VI, Tallant TC, Strom E, Gleiberman AS, Gupta D, et al. An agonist of toll-like receptor 5 has radioprotective activity in mouse and primate models. Science. 2008;**320**:226-230. DOI: 10.1126/science.1154986

[33] Anscher MS, Thrasher B, Rabbani Z, Teicher B, Vujaskovic Z. Antitransforming growth factor-beta antibody 1D11 ameliorates normal tissue damage caused by high-dose radiation. International Journal of Radiation Oncology, Biology, Physics. 2006;**65**:876-881

[34] Anscher MS, Thrasher B, Zgonjanin L, Rabbani ZN, Corbley MJ, Fu K, et al. Small molecular inhibitor of transforming growth factor-beta protects against development of radiation-induced lung injury. International Journal of Radiation Oncology, Biology, Physics. 2008;**71**:829-837. DOI: 10.1016/j.ijrobp.2008.02.046

[35] Massague J. TGF beta in cancer. Cell. 2008;**134**:215-230. DOI: 10.1016/j.cell.2008.07.001

[36] Abdel-Mageed AS, Senagore AJ, Pietryga DW, Connors RH, Giambernardi TA, Hay RV, et al. Intravenous administration of mesenchymal stem cells genetically modified with extracellular superoxide dismutase improves survival in irradiated mice. Blood. 2009;**113**:1201-1203. DOI: 10.1182/blood-2008-07-170936

[37] Saha S, Bhanja P, Kabarriti R, Liu L, Alfieri AA, Guha C. Bone marrow stromal cell transplantation mitigates radiation-induced gastrointestinal syndrome in mice. PLoS ONE. 2011;**6**:e24072. DOI: 10.1371/journal.pone.0024072

[38] Singh VK, Christensen J, Fatanmi OO, Gille D, Ducey EJ, Wise SY, et al. Myeloid progenitors: A radiation countermeasure that is effective when initiated days after irradiation. Radiation Research. 2012;**177**:781-791

[39] Singh VK, Brown DS, Kao TC, Seed TM. Preclinical development of a bridging therapy for radiation casualties. Experimental Hematology. 2010;**38**:61-70. DOI: 10.1016/j.exphem.2009.10.008

[40] Rosen EM, Day R, Singh VK. New approaches to radiation protection. Frontiers in Oncology. 2014;**4**:381. DOI: 10.3389/fonc.2014.00381

[41] Chin MS, Freniere BB, Bonney CF, Lancerotto L, Saleeby JH, Lo YC, et al. Skin perfusion and oxygenation changes in radiation fibrosis. Plastic and Reconstructive Surgery. 2013;**131**:707-716. DOI: 10.1097/PRS.0b013e3182818b94

[42] Chin MS, Freniere BB, Lo YC, Saleeby JH, Baker SP, Strom HM, et al. Hyperspectral imaging for early detection of oxygenation and perfusion changes in irradiated skin. Journal of Biomedical Optics. 2012;**17**:026010. DOI: 10.1117/1.JBO.17.2.026010

[43] Zakeri K, Narayanan D, Vikram B, Evans G, Coleman CN, Prasanna PGS. Decreasing the toxicity of

radiation therapy: Radioprotectors and radiomitigators being developed by the National Cancer Institute through Small Business Innovation Research contracts. International Journal of Radiation Oncology, Biology, Physics. 2019;**104**:188-196. DOI: 10.1016/j.ijrobp.2018.12.027

Chapter 5

Vascular Trauma

Krzysztof Szaniewski, Tomasz Byrczek and Tomasz Sikora

Abstract

Trauma is a leading cause of death and disability in young adults in developed countries with the high impact on future patient quality of life and productivity. The traumatic injury of the vessels is one of the most dangerous types of injury, requiring a fast and reliable diagnosis and, in vast majority of cases, immediate surgical treatment. In this chapter, the authors describe various types of vascular injuries according to injury types and locations. The prehospital care algorithms in patients with vascular trauma are proposed with the emphasis on bleeding control techniques and transportation technique to the nearest hospital. In the next subsection, the various peripheral vascular injuries of specific body areas are described. The truncal vessel trauma is discussed in the next subsection, focusing on fast diagnosis and decision on surgery. In the last subsection, a problem of iatrogenic vascular injury is described due to a rapid increase of minimally invasive techniques in which a vascular injury, as a complication of therapy, may occur.

Keywords: vascular trauma, vascular injury, peripheral vessels injury, truncal vessels injury, iatrogenic vascular trauma, aortic injury

1. Introduction

Trauma has become a leading cause of death among young adults in industrialized nations. In the United States in 2010, trauma was the cause of death in 63% of patients aged 1–24 years and 42% of the patients in the ages 25–44. Furthermore, trauma results with lowered patient's productivity with high economic impact. A vascular trauma incidence is estimated between 1.6 and 2% in adults during peace and between 6 and 12% during war. Most of the civilian casualties are injured by penetrating objects like firearm bullets, blades, or machine parts. In Europe, where access to firearms is limited, most of the penetrating vascular injuries result from criminal acts (e.g., knife stabbing), traffic, and labor accidents [1, 2].

2. Prehospital care in patients with vascular injury

2.1 On-site emergency procedures and medical transport

Fast initial diagnosis, patient's vital signs stabilization together with effective bleeding control, and quick transport to the hospital are crucial factors influencing future prognosis.

After the evaluation of the overall security condition on trauma site (traffic accident, disaster site, explosion area), it is important to predetermine a possible trauma mechanism in order to predict possible vascular injury as well as collateral damage of the adjacent tissues [2].

The next step is the patient examination. After the initial evaluation of vital signs and recording the state of a victim's consciousness (GCS), a CABC rule should be applied (**Table 1**).

After CABC, a trauma extent assessment as well as medical examination are performed (SAMPLE) (**Table 2**). The medical examination should cover all body areas in direction from head to toe including the patient's back and extremities. The aim of that procedure is to find any eventual collateral damage which can be life-threatening. The additional information from other victims or witnesses should be gathered, if possible [3].

After the finishing of medical examination, the patient should be qualified to one of the following groups:

1. LOAD & GO—victim in extremely severe condition. Only a basic set of medical procedures is performed necessary to support life. The transport has a priority [4].

2. STAY & PLAY—all necessary procedures may be performed on-site. The transport follows the initial care.

During the transportation, especially with unstable patient in severe condition, the information to the admitting center (ATMIST scheme) should be sent (**Table 3**) [5].

The portable ultrasound devices are helpful in fast initial diagnosis of the injuries of large vessels of the chest or abdomen with the use of eFAST protocol (chest, pericardium, and abdomen) [6].

Below we propose a procedure of prehospital care in vascular trauma:

1. Initial examination, CABC, SAMPLE

2. Control of the visible external bleeding

3. Evaluation of possible internal bleeding(s)

4. Intravenous access (intramedullar), fluid supply, hypovolemic shock treatment

5. Bleeding control specific to the vascular injury area

6. Medical transport and ATMIST

2.2 Specific procedures of bleeding control according to area of the injury

Vascular injury of the extremities:

- Direct wound compression.

C	Control bleeding—the bleeding controls a visible and life-threatening hemorrhage
A	Airways—secure the airways and evaluate possible obturation causes
B	Breathe—ventilation rate, volume, and effectiveness
C	Circulation—central and peripheral circulation assessment, blood pressure, capillary flow, and skin perfusion

Table 1.
CABC rule in prehospital care of the patient.

S	Symptoms (bleeding, ischemia, shock, fractures, wounds, etc.)
A	Allergies (drugs, food, chemicals (e.g., disinfectants), materials (plaster dressing, etc.))
M	Medicines—recently used or prescribed medicines
P	Past—medical history and pregnancies
L	Lunch—last meal, time, and volume
E	Event—what has happened

Table 2.
SAMPLE rule in the examination of the victim of an accident.

A	Age
T	Time of the event
M	Mechanism
I	Injuries
S	Symptoms
T	Treatment (already performed)

Table 3.
ATMIST algorithm.

- Limb elevation.

  ○ Compression dressing.

- Tourniquet: usually applied on arm or thigh, less often in distal areas (forearm, below the knee) usually 8 cm above the suspected vascular lesion. An effective modification of that technique is to apply two tourniquets, one high on the limb and the second 8 cm above the wound. Then the first one is released, while the second stays closed [3, 7].

- Packing of the bottom of the wound with sterile gauze with continuous compression.

- Hemostatic dressings and substances: in the form of dressing, powder or foam—usually a 3–5 min time is needed to initiate coagulation between a dressing and injury site [3, 8].

Vascular injuries in the connection areas (armpits, groins):

- Direct compression.

- Compression dressing.

- Specific compression systems.

  ○ JETT (Junctional Emergency Treatment Tool).

  ○ SAM Junctional Tourniquet: the systems which are applied on inguinal or axillary regions where traditional compression system application is limited [9, 10].

Neck vasculature lesions:

- Direct compression.
- Compression with contralateral hand.
- Hemostatic media.

Vascular injuries of the head:

- Direct compression.
- Haemostatic suture of the skin vessels.

Vascular injury of the chest:

- Direct compression.
- Occlusive dressing.
- Emergency thoracotomy.

Vascular injury of the abdomen:

- Occlusive dressing.
- Hemostatic foams
  - Abdominal aortic and junctional tourniquet (AAJT)
  - Resuscitative endovascular balloon occlusion of the aorta (REBOA) [11, 12]

Vascular injury of the pelvis:

- Pelvic belt.
- Hemostatic foams.

2.3 Hypovolemic shock and fluid therapy

Patients in hypovolemic shock with controlled external bleeding should be administered with 500–1000 ml of crystalloids, with a constant blood pressure control. Blood pressure may be maintained near to normal values. In patients where there is no possibility to control the external or internal bleeding, crystalloids volume should allow to maintain the systolic blood pressure on the perfusion level (80–90 mmHg) to prevent anaerobic metabolism in supplied tissue. Exceptionally in patients with the traumatic lesion of the central nervous system, the systolic blood pressure should be maintained on higher levels of 100–110 mmHg, which secures cerebral perfusion pressure on the level of 60 mmHg [13].

3. Peripheral vascular injury

Isolated vascular injury of the extremities is the most common vascular injury type during the peace in high-volume trauma center in Europe. The incidence rises in highly urbanized area due to traffic and labor accidents and varies between 1 and 2% of total number of traumatic patients admitted to the ER [14]. In our center, the incidence of the vascular trauma among all traumatic patients was 3% in a 5-year period (2014–2018). In the upper limbs, the regions of elevated risk are the armpit, the medial part of the arm, and the ulnar fossa due to a superficial position of the vascular structures. In the lower limb, attention should be focused on injuries of the groin, the medial thigh area, and the popliteal fossa. The ligation of the artery in vascular injury below the brachial bifurcation or knee trifurcation usually has no risk of the peripheral limb ischemia.

The vascular damage may be caused by penetrating object (like knife blade, a part of a machinery, steel rod, etc.) or may have been an effect of the blunt trauma with the force acting directly on the vessel wall or by the surrounding tissues like bone fragments or luxated joints. Penetrating injuries, mostly with low energy character, constitute 70–90% of cases [15]. Blunt vascular trauma may be the effect of the vessel contusion and secondary thrombosis, which is often a result of the knee joint or upper arm luxation and dislocation of the humerus/tibia causing the blunt trauma.

According to an extent of the wound, in penetrating vascular injury, various clinical manifestations may occur, from puncture wound with minimal bleeding and minute signs of the peripheral ischemia to a large laceration of the skin with life-threatening hemorrhage.

3.1 Diagnosis

The on-site evaluation and diagnosis was described earlier in this chapter; in hospital, the physician after gathering information from the medical emergency service team should also try to obtain information from the patient especially about the traumatic mechanism and possible time of eventual ischemia. The mechanism of injury has a prognostic value. High-energy injuries (penetrating or blunt) have elevated risk of vascular damage, and the risk of amputation is higher in high-energy blunt trauma. Collateral damage of surrounding tissues and adjacent structures may require separate intervention (e.g., orthopedic surgery), or in the case of extensive polytrauma, complex interdisciplinary approach with advanced life support techniques.

It is generally agreed that after 6 hours of the limb ischemia, irreversible changes occur in the nervous and musculatory systems, though it is important to precisely evaluate the onset time. The time may be counted from the injury time or if the ischemic process is iatrogenic (e.g., tourniquet, pressure dressing) from the time in which the blood flow was stopped.

Concomitant diseases and patient's medical history are also important (arteriosclerosis, cardiac diseases, diabetes), as well as medications are prescribed, especially ASA and VKA.

3.2 Medical examination

The decision of immediate surgery, especially when active bleeding is concerned, is crucial at the first minutes of examination, due to a high mortality rate in the case of misdiagnosis. A vast majority of victims presenting "hard signs" of vascular trauma require an immediate operation with sensitivity above 90%; on the other hand, if no "hard sign" is present (**Table 4**) (**Figures 1** and **2**), the vascular trauma probability is very low [16].

"Soft signs" are not so specific in the prediction of the vascular injuries, and immediate open repair usually is not necessary. A single soft sign increases a chance

Hard signs	Soft signs
Active pulsatile bleeding	Pulse deficit
Rapidly expanding hematoma	Neurological deficit
Pulselessness	Paleness of the extremity
Acute ischemia	Nonexpanding hematoma
Vascular thrill	—
Bruit	—

Table 4.
Hard and soft signs of vascular trauma.

of vascular injury in 10%, and two or more soft signs can have a vascular injury rate of 25% [17, 18] (**Figure 1**).

The pulse and extremity blood supply should be evaluated in the first place. A physical examination and the pulse palpation of **all extremities** should be performed.

The bleeding should be stopped as soon as possible by the use of compression dressing and tourniquet or if the situation allows temporary shunting of the damaged artery or vein. The vessel clamping or ligation can be done only in the last resort, when the patient's life is directly at risk. If the damaged vessel is clearly visible and ischaemic symptoms occur, the patient should be referred to vascular surgery in order to perform emergency revascularization. After the bleeding control, the focus should be directed on the chances of the limb salvage. The MESS score is the most popular tool in assessment of the extremity salvage chance [cite

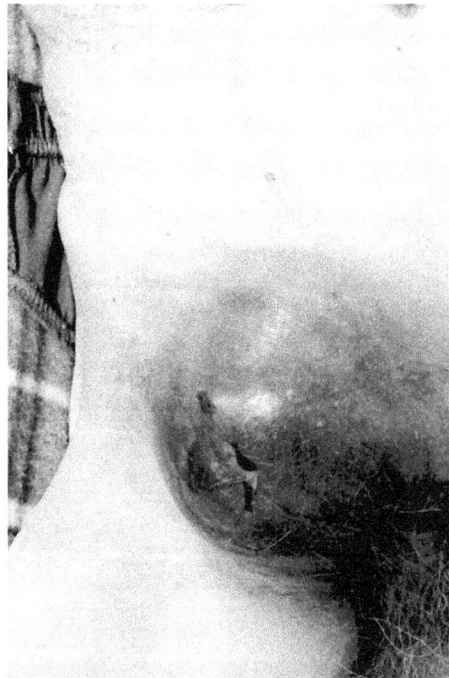

Figure 1.
A typical "hard sign" of the blunt vascular injury of the groin.

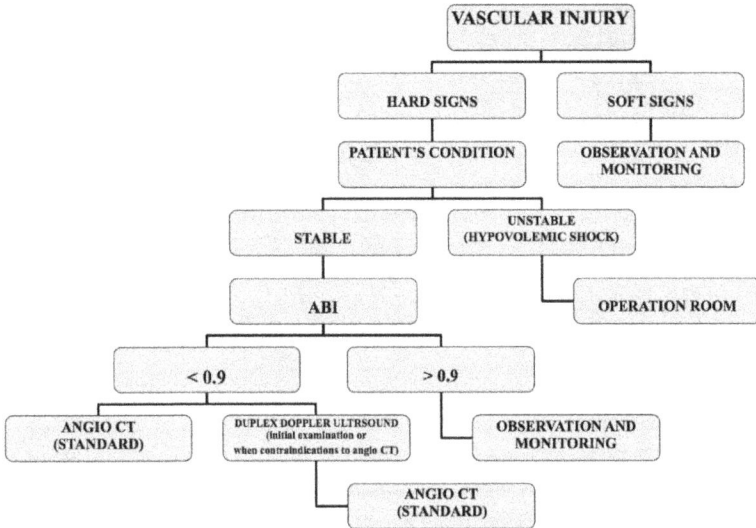

Figure 2.
The algorithm of the management of the peripheral vascular injury patient.

mess]. Afterwards, if ischaemic signs are present, the limb condition should be rated according to TASC II categorization. Quite often there is no sign of active bleeding, especially in young patients where even a total intersection of femoral or brachial artery does not end with massive hemorrhage due to a vessel end contraction and thrombosis [18–20].

Ankle-brachial index (ABI) or arterial pressure index (API) is a useful adjunct to physical examination. ABI value <0.9 has 87% sensitivity and 97% specificity in the assessment of vascular trauma, reaching 95% of sensitivity when focused on big arterial trunks. ABI value below 0.9 is an direct indication for further imaging as US, CT angiography, or MRI. On the other hand, ABI value >0.9 with no signs of the orthopedic injury allows to release the patient from ER, with the further referral to outpatient clinic in the next few days for reassessment of eventual delayed presentation of vascular injury [21].

3.3 Treatment

In the first option of treatment, especially in patients presenting with TASC II and III category , the treatment of choice is an open repair. Both stumps of the damaged vessels should be identified and clamped.

After the thrombectomy and vessel stump preparation, an anastomosis is performed. The best option is end-to-end anastomosis without any conduit; however that option is only possible in directly cut vessels where the surgeon is able to mobilize vessel stumps from the surrounding tissue very often soaked with the blood and tissue liquids. If there is any tension between arterial or venous stumps, the better option is to make a conduit, preferably from autologous vein. Reversed great saphenous vein (GSV) graft is the most popular choice; however, there are other possibilities like small saphenous vein and basilic or radio-cephalic vein. However, SSV and other peripheral veins are more difficult to harvest and may have insufficient diameter.

If the vein is not available, the surgeon faces a decision whether to use a homologous material (if available) like frozen bovine graft or frozen homograft

Surgical material
Autologous vein GSV, SSV, RCV, BV
Frozen bovine graft
Homograft
Silver-coated prosthesis (Braun, Intergard)
PTFE
Rifampin-soaked Dacron

Table 5.
Material for grafting in vascular injury.

or to use synthetic prosthesis. If the synthetic prosthesis has to be used as a conduit, the most infection-resistant option available on shelf should be utilized (**Table 5**).

The endovascular modality is limited only to cases with preserved continuity of the vessel, which can be visualized only in CT angiography, and we recommend that option to patients with TASC I category (viable limb). Usually endovascular approach is effective in arterial puncture with pseudoaneurysm formation or arterial thrombosis in cases of isolated blunt trauma mostly in popliteal and axial region or in cases of arm luxation (**Figures 3–5**).

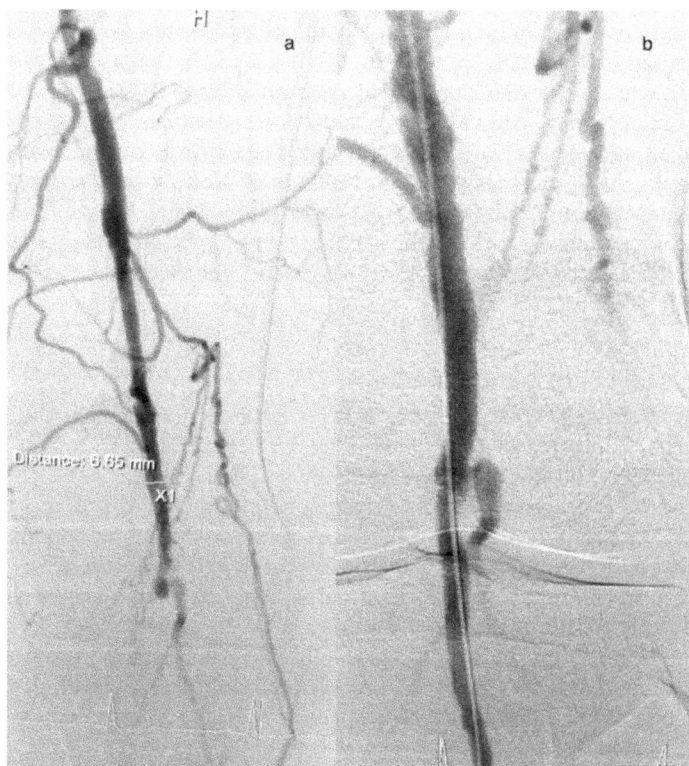

Figure 3.
Blunt trauma of the popliteal fossa resolved by the endovascular approach. (a) thrombosis of the popliteal artery, (b) restored flow in the vessel

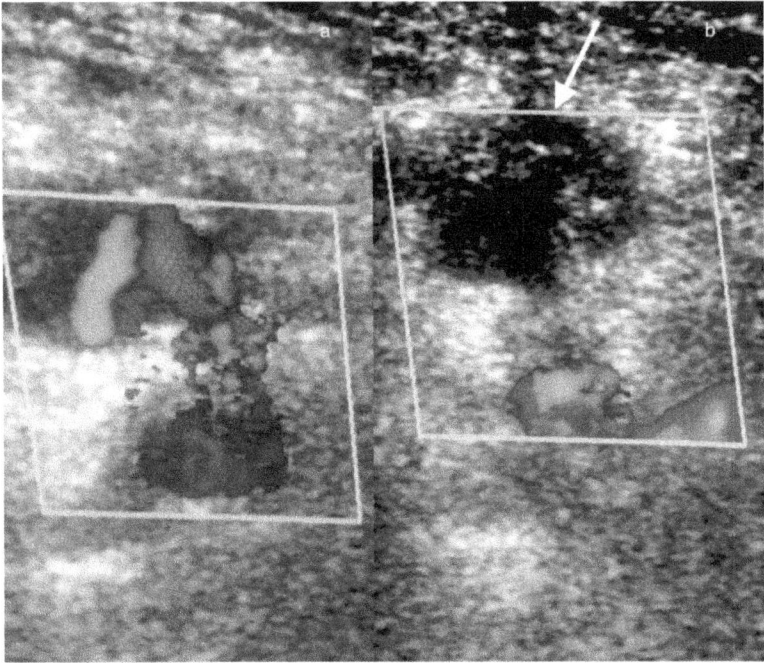

Figure 4.
The pseudoaneurysm sac successfully closed by biothrombin injection (arrow) [22].

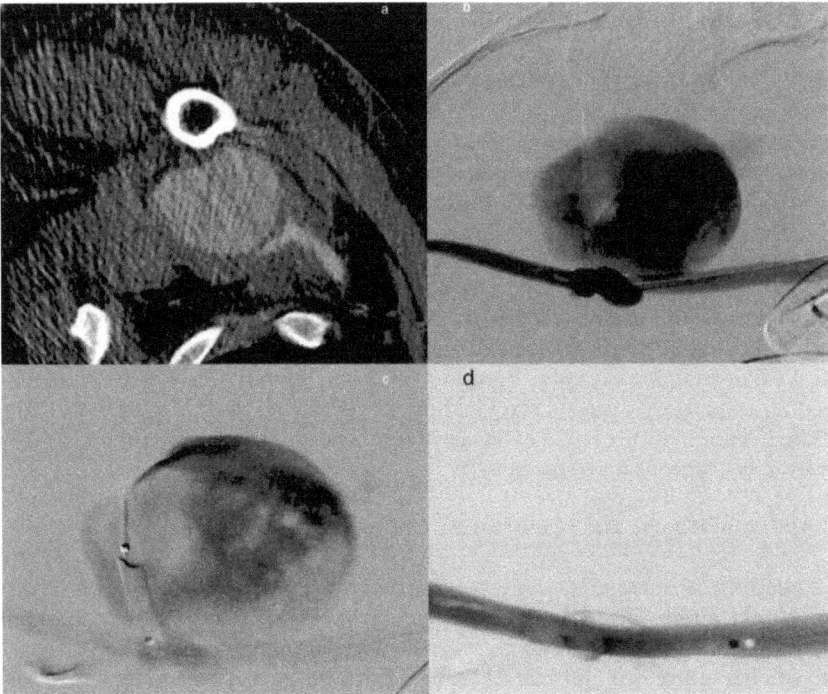

Figure 5.
The pseudoaneurysm of the right axillary artery successfully resolved by trans-catheter thrombin injection. (a) a CT scan of the lesion, (b) arteriography image of the lesion before the injection, (c) a balloon catheter occluding the aneurysm "jet", (d) angiographic image of the axillary artery after the treatment [22].

4. Truncal large vessels trauma

4.1 Thoracic aorta injury

The traumatic damage of the thoracic aorta is usually an effect of traffic accidents or sudden fall resulting from acceleration-deceleration mechanisms. Less often it is a result of the penetrating injury like knife stabbing or gunshot. In that case the damage of the aortic wall is usually complete with massive hemorrhage into mediastinum or pleural cavity, which is in most cases fatal. In blunt trauma, the most common site of injury is the descending aorta left from subclavian artery ostium and below the aortic ligament. In most cases, the intimal tear occurs resulting in acute dissection progressing downwards to the visceral arteries and to the aortic bifurcation. Sometimes we can observe almost complete aortic wall tear, pseudoaneurysm formation in the chest and progressing dissection.

The computed angiotomography is a routine examination which allows to diagnose the thoracic aorta injury with high accuracy and has become a standard procedure in chest injuries. If there is no possibility of CT scanning, a transesophageal ultrasound can be used however in a very limited fashion.

From the beginning of the century, a thoracic endovascular stent-graft implantation (TEVAR) has become a routine procedure in salvaging patients with aortic injury, decreasing a perioperative mortality from 70% to 15–30%. If open surgical procedure has to be performed, a chance of survival drops dramatically to 15–20%. The open repair usually requires high aortic clamping, and the risk of the neurological deficit resulting from spinal cord ischemia is significantly higher than during the TEVAR. In TEVAR, however, the risk of spinal cord ischemia is also significant (23%), especially in cases when the graft fabric covers the ostium of the left subclavian artery (LSA) and suppresses the collateral circulation from internal mammary artery (LIMA) to the intercostals. If the patient is in stable condition, a surgeon can bypass the left subclavian ostium, by performing a carotid-subclavian conduit preserving the flow in LSA and LIMA. Another popular neuroprotective option is the drainage of the cerebrospinal fluid to reduce the pressure from eventual spine edema. In many centers that procedure is performed routinely during TEVAR or open repair when LSA closure is necessary [4, 23, 24].

4.2 Large veins of the chest

The rupture of the large veins in the chest is usually fatal, and patients do no reach the hospital. However, if the patient's condition allows for medial thoracotomy with sternotomy to expose superior vena cava, there is a chance to control the bleeding and after the patient stabilization to reconstruct the damaged vessel. There are some reports of successful endovascular treatment of vena cava injury [25–27]; however all concern iatrogenic injuries.

4.3 Abdominal aorta and iliac arteries

Abdominal aorta injuries result more often from penetrating mechanism than from blunt trauma. The location of the vessel makes it relatively resistant for blunt injury. If blunt aortic injury occurs, it is usually a part of extensive polytrauma with spine fracture and multiple adjacent organ damage. An exception may be an abdominal aortic rupture during blunt trauma of the abdomen without any collateral damage, which can occur during a car accident or a fall. More frequent are penetrating injures being a result of a criminal act or labor accident. The patient usually presents symptoms of hypovolemic shock, and the first steps should be done to stabilize the vital signs and blood pressure and secure the adequate volume of blood and plasma. The CT scan is a standard procedure confirming an initial diagnosis with visible hematoma in retroperitoneal space. The REBOA procedure (**Figure 6**) is useful during patient stabilization and preparation to surgery or endovascular repair. In open repair a medial abdominal access is used to expose the aorta for clamping and vascular reconstruction usually by the use of polyester or PTFE graft [28]. Less often a simple suture of patch from polyester or autologous vein is used. If there is additional collateral damage like intestine tear, hepatic or renal injury or pelvic fracture, it can be done simultaneously. In cases of isolated aortic damage, usually resulting from penetrating mechanism, an endovascular stent-graft implantation (EVAR) is an effective option.

Blunt iliac artery injuries usually result in pelvic polytrauma with multiple fractures of the pelvis and possible damage of the bladder, uterus, intestines and ureter. In most cases an interdisciplinary approach of specialized trauma team is necessary, and a vascular surgeon's job is to restore the blood flow stopped by thrombosis of the iliac artery or to stop the bleeding and to perform the vascular reconstruction. In cases of hypogastric artery injury, the vessel ligation is the most common solution. In common iliac artery or external iliac artery injury, a reconstruction with the use of artificial bypass is the first choice. The venous grafting has a limited application due to not sufficient diameters of available veins. In cases in which an infection risk is elevated, silver knitted grafts are the most popular option. The isolated blunt external

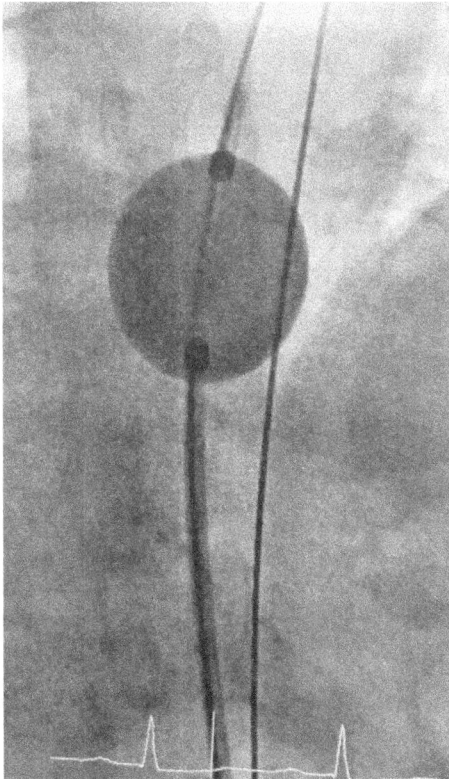

Figure 6.
REBOA technique in salvaging the patient with an aortic rupture.

iliac artery above the inguinal ligament resulting in its thrombosis and chronic limb ischemia in young patients resulting from a bike accident were reported [29].

Penetrating external iliac artery injuries especially in the region of inguinal ligament, known as death triangle injury, are challenging cases where fast decision of surgery is life-saving. The bleeding control in that region is difficult and possible only by direct compression or by modified REBOA procedure when the balloon is opened in the common iliac artery. The open repair is a gold standard because most of the injuries result from a knife stabbing or gunshot, and endovascular endografting has a limited application.

4.4 The injury of the inferior vena cava and iliac veins

A penetrating injury of the inferior vena cava usually produces a large retroperitoneal hematoma having a tendency to self-cease with the drop of the blood pressure and compression produced by the hematoma. That condition is however unstable, and the patient may die suddenly among the symptoms of irreversible hypovolemic shock. Urgent surgical exploration is necessary to seal the rupture in the vein wall. As much as possible the VCI should be exposed to find the rupture, and after the compression of the inflow and outflow site, suture it or reconstruct by the use of artificial graft (usually PTFE). Recently, there have been reports of successful treatment of the VCI ruptures by the use of covered stents or stent grafts however in majority concerning iatrogenic damage [14, 30–33].

The blunt injury of IVC is a very rare condition, with a prevalence of 1% of all blunt abdominal traumas resulting in dissection, pseudoaneurysm formation, or IVC thrombosis. In the literature there are single reports in the management of IVS blunt injuries usually catheter-directed techniques [16, 34, 35].

4.5 The injury of the carotid arteries and jugular vein

The penetrating injuries of the carotid arteries and jugular veins are mostly resulting in a stabbing effect or an effect of the gunshot. The bleeding control in the case of open wound of the neck is a crucial element of the further success. In the case of the venous injury, a direct compression on the ruptured vessel is usually sufficient to transport the patient to the operation room and to perform exploration and vessel reconstruction. The problem occurs in the case of arterial damage with high-volume blood outflow. Too much compression may lead to severe neurological deficits so pressure should be administered only to stop the bleeding. Additional wound packing may also be helpful. In our opinion every penetrating vascular injury of the neck should be surgically explored in order to prevent a secondary damage as uncontrolled hematoma expansion leading to neurological and respiratory deficits which is supported by the data from the literature [36, 37]. The unstable patients are qualified to immediate surgery, while the stable ones after fast-track imaging in order to localize the exact lesion location should also undergo surgical exploration (**Figure 7**).

Blunt injury of the cervical vessels is a relatively rare condition with prevalence <0.1% and however related to increased mortality and morbidity due to a cerebral infarction. The symptoms of the cerebral ischemia may occur up to 72 h after an accident due to an embolisation from the local vessel thrombosis or dissection. The CT angiography scans should be performed in all patients suffering the injury of the neck in stable condition without signs of rapidly developing hematoma in order to exclude a sub-intimal dissection or thrombosis which can be a source of embolic material. In these patients an endovascular option is a good solution for covering a damaged area with a closed cell stent or stent-graft.

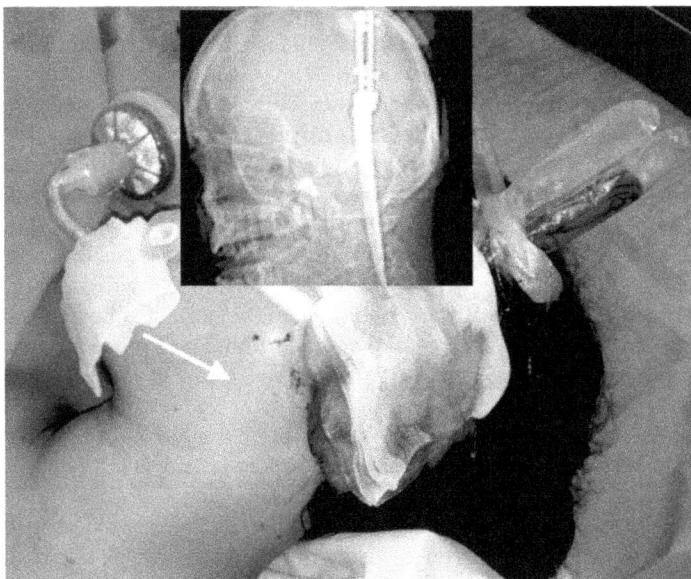

Figure 7.
Left carotid artery injury with the compressing hematoma (arrow).

5. Iatrogenic vascular injury

In the recent years, in the development of mini-invasive and endovascular techniques, an increase of iatrogenic vascular injuries is observed. A most common complication of the vascular access in endovascular approach is hematoma and pseudoaneurysm in the access site [22, 38]. The rate of these incidents varies between 0.5 and 1.0% and recently was decreased by the use of various vascular sealing systems. A perforation or tear of the arterial wall not in the access site is the second very frequent complication of the endovascular procedure. The typical location of the perforation is iliac arteries, when during the approach to the target lesion (coronary arteries, carotid arteries, abdominal aorta) a hydrophilic guidewire perforates the vessel typically in the location of arteriosclerotic plaque [5, 39]. If the guidewire perforation is noticed quickly, usually it has no consequences besides small extravasation which may require a low-pressure balloon inflation to seal the leak. Sometimes, however, the perforation is not noticed, and some larger bore devices (balloons, stent-graft parts) may be pushed outside the arteries producing a large diameter tear in the arterial wall. If there is no possibility to seal the leak by the use of stent-graft, the only solution is to open the low-pressure balloon inside the vessel and urgent laparotomy or thoracotomy.

In open repair, the iatrogenic traumatic vascular trauma has been observed mostly during orthopedic repositions, general surgery procedures, gynecology, and neurosurgery. After an introduction of the laparoscopic techniques at the beginning of the last decade of the XX century, an incidence of unintentional rupture of the large vessels in abdominal and pelvic region during the introduction of the trocars increased. That type of the injury may have very dramatic outcome, with massive and rapidly increasing hematoma especially when the abdominal part of vena cava or iliac veins are concerned. In that case only an instant conversion and pressure packing may stop the bleeding and save the patient. After a bleeding control is achieved, the vascular reconstruction may take place which is very often limited to pacing a vascular suture on the vein; less frequently the patch, bypass or ligation is needed [40–42].

When arterial vessels are damaged, a massive bleeding is not so often; in some cases, one can observe a pseudoaneurysm formation, vessel thrombosis, or retroperitoneal hematoma which also requires an urgent surgery; however, the symptoms are not so dramatic and chances are better. In that case, a vascular reconstruction usually ends with suturing the damaged artery. Sometimes, a thrombectomy is performed, with more extensive reconstructions with patches or bypasses. In the pelvic region, when hypogastric artery is damaged, very often a ligation of the vessel is one of the options.

Injuries of the hepatic arteries or vascular structures of hepatic ligament are less frequent and cause mostly by thermal mechanism during electrocoagulation [43].

Vascular injury during the orthopedic surgery is not a frequent complication with an incidence of 0.05–0.1%. However due to a large number of procedures performed, it concerns patients in almost every hospital in which total hip and knee arthroplasty is performed, as well as urgent repositions of the spine and long bones of the extremities with stabilization by the use of external or internal material [44, 45]. During the hip or knee replacement, the mechanism of injury is usually indirect, resulting from torsion and elongation forces resulting in intimal tear and vessel thrombosis. In rare cases the misplaced fixation screws of the acetabulum caused active bleeding or thrombosis of external iliac artery. During the open repositions, the mechanism is usually directly caused by a stabilization material and fixation screws resulting in arterial damage. In that case, the time of diagnosis is crucial, especially when iliac, femoral, or brachial arteries are involved. In some cases like popliteal artery thrombosis after a total knee replacement, an endovascular option is possible. However, in most cases, an arterial reconstruction is the only possible solution. Repositions of the bones of forearm and below the knee have a significantly lower risk of ischaemic complication due to the anatomic reasons, but an active bleeding or pseudoaneurysms may occur. In that area, however, a ligation of the single main arterial trunk like radial or tibial artery usually has no ischaemic consequences.

6. Conclusions

Vascular injuries are not a frequent condition; however, they are one of the most dangerous and challenging cases for medical personnel in the field of proper diagnostics and therapy. In the vast majority of cases, regardless of whether they concern civilian or warfare victims, there are penetrating injuries resulting in massive bleeding or limb-threatening ischemia. The implementation of proper treatment already at the prehospital stage is an essential factor for the patient survival and the limb salvage.

Fast initial assessment of the patient's condition based on the CABC algorithm, adopting an appropriate transport strategy (Load & Go or Stay & Play), application of bleeding control techniques adequate to the area of injury, and early prevention of hypovolemic shock are the key factors for prehospital treatment.

Due to the rapid development of minimally invasive techniques in various fields of medicine (cardiology, neurology, abdominal surgery, urology), the number of iatrogenic vascular injuries increased. Despite the low incidence of such events, iatrogenic injuries are quite common due to high volumes of minimally invasive procedures performed and require the involvement of a vascular surgeon.

The vascular trauma is very often a part of polytrauma requiring the interdisciplinary trauma team of various specialists to perform a wide range of operations in one time such as vascular reconstructions together with reconstructive orthopedics or reconstruction of the urinary tract. The vascular trauma patients and especially patients with polytrauma should be transported to specialized trauma centers with the high reference level.

Vascular Trauma
DOI: http://dx.doi.org/10.5772/intechopen.88285

Author details

Krzysztof Szaniewski*, Tomasz Byrczek and Tomasz Sikora
Department of Vascular Surgery and Emergency Department, Trauma Center,
St. Barbara Hospital, Sosnowiec, Poland

*Address all correspondence to: kszaniewski@gmail.com

IntechOpen

References

[1] Sidawy AN, Perler BA. Rutherford's Vascular Surgery and Endovascular Therapy. 9th ed. Philadelphia, PA: Elsevier; 2019

[2] Hoff WS, Holevar M, Nagy KK, Patterson L, Young JS, Arrillaga A, et al. Practice management guidelines for the evaluation of blunt abdominal trauma: The East practice management guidelines work group. The Journal of Trauma. 2002;**53**(3):602-615

[3] Guła P, Machała W, Wydawnictwo Lekarskie PZWL. Postępowanie w obrażeniach ciała w praktyce SOR. Warszawa: Wydawnictwo Lekarskie PZWL; 2017

[4] Akhmerov A, DuBose J, Azizzadeh A. Blunt thoracic aortic injury: Current therapies, outcomes, and challenges. Annals of Vascular Diseases. 2019;**12**(1):1-5

[5] Mehta V, Pandit BN, Mehra P, Nigam A, Vyas A, Yusuf J, et al. Massive bleeding from guidewire perforation of an external iliac artery: Treatment with hand-made stent-graft placement. Cardiovascular and Interventional Radiology. 2016;**39**(1):106-110

[6] Sosada K, Żurawiński W, Wydawnictwo Lekarskie PZWL. Ostre stany zagrożenia życia w obrażeniach ciała. Warszawa: PZWL Wydawnictwo Lekarskie; 2018

[7] Davidovic LB, Cinara IS, Ille T, Kostic DM, Dragas MV, Markovic DM. Civil and war peripheral arterial trauma: review of risk factors associated with limb loss. Vascular. 2005;**13**(3):141-147

[8] Prichayudh S, Rassamee P, Sriussadaporn S, Pak-Art R, Sriussadaporn S, Kritayakirana K, et al. Abdominal vascular injuries: Blunt vs. penetrating. Injury. 2019;**50**(1):137-141

[9] Johnson JE, Sims RK, Hamilton DJ, Kragh JF. Safety and effectiveness evidence of SAM(r) junctional tourniquet to control inguinal hemorrhage in a perfused cadaver model. Journal of Special Operations Medicine: A Peer Reviewed Journal for SOF Medical Professionals. 2014;**14**(2):21-25

[10] Smith S, White J, Wanis KN, Beckett A, McAlister VC, Hilsden R. The effectiveness of junctional tourniquets: A systematic review and meta-analysis. Journal of Trauma and Acute Care Surgery. 2019;**86**(3):532-539

[11] Coleman JJ, Zarzaur BL. Surgical management of abdominal trauma. The Surgical Clinics of North America. 2017;**97**(5):1107-1117

[12] Trellopoulos G, Georgiadis GS, Aslanidou EA, Nikolopoulos ES, Pitta X, Papachristodoulou A, et al. Endovascular management of peripheral arterial trauma in patients presenting in hemorrhagic shock. The Journal of Cardiovascular Surgery. 2012;**53**(4):495-506

[13] Malgras B, Prunet B, Lesaffre X, Boddaert G, Travers S, Cungi P-J, et al. Damage control: Concept and implementation. Journal of Visceral Surgery. 2017;**154**(Suppl 1):S19-S29

[14] Branco BC, Musonza T, Long MA, Chung J, Todd SR, Wall MJ, et al. Survival trends after inferior vena cava and aortic injuries in the United States. Journal of Vascular Surgery. 2018;**68**(6):1880-1888

[15] Badole C, Patond K, Mk K. Salvage versus amputation: Utility of mangled extremity severity score in severely injured lower limbs. Indian Journal of Orthopaedics. 2007;**41**(3):183

[16] Cheaito A, Tillou A, Lewis C, Cryer H. Management of traumatic blunt IVC injury. International Journal of Surgery Case Reports. 2016;**28**:26-30

[17] Brunner MP, Cronin EM, Wazni O, Baranowski B, Saliba WI, Sabik JF, et al. Outcomes of patients requiring emergent surgical or endovascular intervention for catastrophic complications during transvenous lead extraction. Heart Rhythm. 2014;**11**(3):419-425

[18] Johansen K, Daines M, Howey T, Helfet D, Hansen ST. Objective criteria accurately predict amputation following lower extremity trauma. The Journal of Trauma. 1990;**30**(5):568-572-573

[19] Loja MN, Sammann A, DuBose J, Li C-S, Liu Y, Savage S, et al. The mangled extremity score and amputation: Time for a revision. Journal of Trauma and Acute Care Surgery. 2017;**82**(3):518-523

[20] Norgren L, Hiatt WR, Dormandy JA, Nehler MR, Harris KA, Fowkes FGR. Inter-society consensus for the management of peripheral arterial disease (TASC II). Journal of Vascular Surgery. 2007;**45**(1):S5-S67

[21] Feliciano DV. Management of peripheral arterial injury. Current Opinion in Critical Care. 2010;**16**(6):602-608

[22] Orawczyk T, Urbanek T, Biolik G, Ziaja D, Szaniewski K, Kuczmik W, et al. Thrombin injection in obliteration of femoral false aneurysms—Own experience. Chirurgia Polska. 2004;**6**(1):7-18

[23] Pang D, Hildebrand D, Bachoo P. Thoracic endovascular repair (TEVAR) versus open surgery for blunt traumatic thoracic aortic injury. In: Cochrane Vascular Group, editor. Cochrane Database Syst Rev. Hoboken, New Jersey, USA: John Wiley & Sons, Ltd; 2019. [cited 2019 Jun 15]; Available from: http://doi.wiley.

com/10.1002/14651858.CD006642.pub3. ISSN: 1465-1858

[24] Son S-A, Jung H, Cho JY, Oh T-H, Do YW, Lim KH, et al. Mid-term outcomes of endovascular repair for traumatic thoracic aortic injury: A single-center experience. European Journal of Trauma and Emergency Surgery. 2019. [cited 2019 June 15]; Available from: http://link.springer. com/10.1007/s00068-019-01166-6

[25] Altuwaijri T, Nouh T, Alburakan A, Altoijry A. Long-term follow-up of endovascular repair of iatrogenic superior vena cava injury: A case report. Medicine (Baltimore). 2018;**97**(50):e13610

[26] Azizzadeh A, Pham MT, Estrera AL, Coogan SM, Safi HJ. Endovascular repair of an iatrogenic superior vena caval injury: A case report. Journal of Vascular Surgery. 2007;**46**(3):569-571

[27] Mattox KL, Feliciano DV, Burch J, Beall AC, Jordan GL, De Bakey ME. Five thousand seven hundred sixty cardiovascular injuries in 4459 patients. Epidemiologic evolution 1958 to 1987. Annals of Surgery. 1989;**209**(6):698-705-707

[28] Weale R, Kong V, Manchev V, Bekker W, Oosthuizen G, Brysiewicz P, et al. Management of intra-abdominal vascular injury in trauma laparotomy: A South African experience. Canadian Journal of Surgery. 2018;**61**(3):158-164

[29] Kazibudzki M, Orawczyk T, Ludyga T, Krupowies A. Cyclist's injury—The cause of symptoms of chronic ischaemia of the lower limb young patients. Chirurgia Polska. 2005;7(4):292-295

[30] Matsumoto S, Jung K, Smith A, Coimbra R. Management of IVC injury: Repair or ligation? A propensity score matching analysis using the national trauma data bank. Journal

of the American College of Surgeons. 2018;**226**(5):752-759.e2

[31] Morishita H, Yamagami T, Matsumoto T, Takeuchi Y, Sato O, Nishimura T. Endovascular repair of a perforation of the vena caval wall caused by the retrieval of a gunther tulip filter after long-term implantation. Cardiovascular and Interventional Radiology. 2011;**34**(S2):321-323

[32] de Naeyer G, Degrieck I. Emergent infrahepatic vena cava stenting for life-threatening perforation. Journal of Vascular Surgery. 2005;**41**(3):552-554

[33] Starzl TE, Kaupp HA, Beheler EM, Freeark RJ. Penetrating injuries of the inferior vena cava. The Surgical Clinics of North America. 1963;**43**:387-400

[34] Kunkala M, Jenkins DH, McEachen J, Stockland A, Zielinski MD. Nonoperative management of traumatic suprahepatic inferior vena cava pseudoaneurysms. Journal of Vascular Surgery. 2011;**54**(6):80S-82S

[35] Sabat J, Hsu C-H, Chu Q, Tan T-W. The mortality for surgical repair is similar to ligation in patients with traumatic portal vein injury. Journal of Vascular Surgery. Venous and Lymphatic Disorders. 2019;7(3):399-404

[36] Nowicki J, Stew B, Ooi E. Penetrating neck injuries: A guide to evaluation and management. Annals of the Royal College of Surgeons of England. 2018;**100**(1):6-11

[37] Rutman AM, Vranic JE, Mossa-Basha M. Imaging and management of blunt cerebrovascular injury. Radiographics. 2018;**38**(2):542-563

[38] Eleshra A, Kim D, Park HS, Lee T. Access site pseudoaneurysms after endovascular intervention for peripheral arterial diseases. Annals of Surgical Treatment and Research. 2019;**96**(6):305-312

[39] Awan MU, Omar B, Qureshi G, Awan GM. Successful treatment of iatrogenic external iliac artery perforation with covered stent: Case report and review of the literature. Cardiology Research. 2017;**8**(5):246-253

[40] Guloglu R, Dilege S, Aksoy M, Alimoglu O, Yavuz N, Mihmanli M, et al. Major retroperitoneal vascular injuries during laparoscopic cholecystectomy and appendectomy. Journal of Laparoendoscopic & Advanced Surgical Techniques. 2004;**14**(2):73-76

[41] Hauser J, Lehnhardt M, Steinau H-U, Homann H-H. Trocar injury of the retroperitoneal vessels followed by life-threatening postischemic compartment syndrome of both lower extremities. Surgical Laparoscopy, Endoscopy & Percutaneous Techniques. 2008;**18**(2):222-224

[42] Li Z, Zhao L, Wang K, Cheng J, Zhao Y, Ren W. Characteristics and treatment of vascular injuries: a review of 387 cases at a Chinese center. International Journal of Clinical and Experimental Medicine. 2014;**7**(12):4710-4719

[43] Gupta V, Gupta V, Joshi P, Kumar S, Kulkarni R, Chopra N, et al. Management of post cholecystectomy vascular injuries. The Surgeon. 2018. [cited 2019 June 17]. Available from: https://linkinghub.elsevier.com/retrieve/pii/S1479666X18301203

[44] Lopera JE, Restrepo CS, Gonzales A, Trimmer CK, Arko F. Aortoiliac vascular injuries after misplacement of fixation screws. Journal of Trauma—Injury, Infection and Critical Care. 2010;**69**(4):870-875

[45] Parvizi J, Pulido L, Slenker N, Macgibeny M, Purtill JJ, Rothman RH. Vascular injuries after total joint arthroplasty. The Journal of Arthroplasty. 2008;**23**(8):1115-1121

Chapter 6

Nail Trauma

Rebeca Astorga Veganzones

Abstract

The nails are important elements of the finger, not only aesthetically, but also for its functionality. Not only to protecting the tip of the finger helps us but also to perform meticulously fine dexterity activities. Due to the high incidence of nail injuries seen in a trauma emergency service, it is essential to know, at least, basic aspects of the anatomy and physiology of the nail and what should be the appropriate treatment based on the injury presented by the patient. Injuries such as subungual hematomas are resolved in short time, however, more complex lesions require minor surgical intervention to obtain good results. In this chapter, additionally to reviewing the anatomy-physiological aspects of the nail, the principles of treatment of nail traumas are detailed.

Keywords: nail anatomy, nail physiology, nail trauma, subungual hematoma, nail surgery

1. Introduction

Although commonly said nail, it is a unit and it is an important element in the distal digit. It is a complex structure that is truly vital to daily life and civilized existence. Fingernails have an important role in hand function, to protect the dorsal surface of the distal phalanges and increase sensitive of the fingertip. Furthermore, the nails facilitate the pinch of small objects and have a cosmetic role.

Fingertip injuries account for 15–24% of all hand injuries, particularly affecting the 4–30-year-old age group [1].

To achieve an optimal outcome, a good initial treatment is necessary because an inadequate or insufficient treatment can derivate in aesthetics and functionality sequels. Hence, to know anatomy and physiology, it is fundamental.

2. Anatomy and physiology of the nail unit

The structural and functional features of the nail unit are unique, clinics and surgeons must understand them thoroughly. Although this chapter discusses each component individually, it is important to understand how the basic structural components of the distal digit interrelate. Abnormality of one of these structures has a profound impact on the other components.

The nail anatomy unit compromises the nail plate, the surrounding soft tissues, and their vasculature and innervation based upon the distal phalanx (**Figure 1**).

2.1 Surrounding soft tissues

Hyponychium: it is the distal limit of the adhesion of the nail plate and it is a histologically specialized area making the transition between the nail bed and pulp

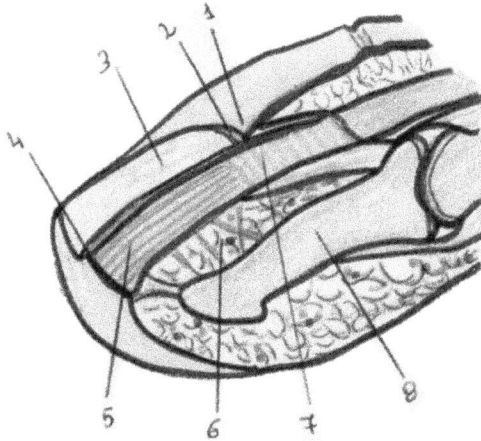

Figure 1.
Nail anatomy: 1. proximal nail fold; 2. eponychium; 3. nail plate; 4. hyponychium; 5. nail bed; 6. subungual subcutaneous; 7. nail matrix; and 8. distal phalanx.

tissue. It has the function as mechanical barrier because prevent accumulation of foreign bodies between the nail plate and the nail bed.

Paronychium: it includes all soft tissues lateral to the nail. The lateral nail folds provide the cushioned cutaneous lateral margins of the nail and is again histologically specialized because protects adjacent nail structures from contamination.

Eponychium: it is a lip of skin that is adherent to the dorsal aspect of the nail plate and conceals all or part of the nail matrix, which is clinically manifest as the "lunula." It combines with the nail plate to provide protective layer over the matrix. This protection extends to blocking from ultraviolet radiation, diminish risk of malignance. Eponychium also combine with the cuticle to provide a seal against irritants and other agents that might disturb matrix function and hence nail growth. So that, remove the cuticle with manicure should be discouraged.

2.2 Nail plate (nail)

The nail plate is only produced by the nail matrix. It is a modified form of stratum corneum cells arranged in successive layers that overlying the nail bed and matrix. Its deep surface is streaked with longitudinal grooves that contribute to fastening it to the underlying nail bed.

It is curved in both longitudinal and transverse axes. This allows it to be embedded in nail folds at its proximal and lateral margins, which provide strong attachment and make the free edge a useful tool.

The tissues beneath the nail plate are divided into nail matrix (15–25%) and the nail bed (75–85%).

Nail matrix or germinative (dorsal matrix), is where the nail-forming epithelial structure. It extends to the distal edge of the lunula, that is the visible distal portion of the conventional matrix as a pale blue-gray half-moon structure emerging from under the proximal nail fold.

Histologically this area has a multilayered epithelium whose duplication is the basic of nail plate formation. The proximal matrix is more productive than distal matrix near to the nail bed.

Nail bed or sterile matrix (ventral matrix), is the tissue that the nail plate rests on and adheres to. It extends from the distal margin of the lunula to the hyponychium and it has a pattern of longitudinal epidermal ridges stretching to the lunula. This part has a low rate of proliferation and complement of keratin expression that lacks the keratins of terminal differentiation seen in normal skin, but this is reversible, and when a nail is avulsed, these keratins are expressed as a nail bed develops the more matt surface of cornified epithelium.

2.3 Vascular supply

2.3.1 Arterial supply

The nail unit is vascularized by the terminal branches of the palmar digital arteries that these are connected by dorsal and palmar arches. There are three arches to blood supply the nail unit, so that, it can survive with extensive damage to the blood supply (**Figure 2**).

The small vessels of the nail bed are orientated in the same axis than the ridges.

2.3.2 Venous drainage

It is by deep and superficial systems. The deep system corresponds to the arterial, and the superficial system exist dorsal and palmar digital veins (**Figure 2**).

2.4 Nerve supply

The distal digits have sensory and autonomic nerves. The sensory nerves are to terminal branches are derived from fine oblique branches of the volar collateral nerves to the second, third and fourth fingers. In the first and fifth digit, there are dorsal collateral nerves that supply the innervation. These branches usually run to the nail folds and pass under the nail bed at the level of the lunula, although there are minor variations.

Autonomic nerves end in fine arborizations where there are special receptors that are essentials for vascular control or two-point discrimination. Clearly, loss of the sensory function or the fingertips greatly impairs all function of the entire hand. Tactile sensory perception is the only or the five sense nor confined to the head, so that, loss of the sensory function of the fingertips is "to render the eyes of the finger blind."

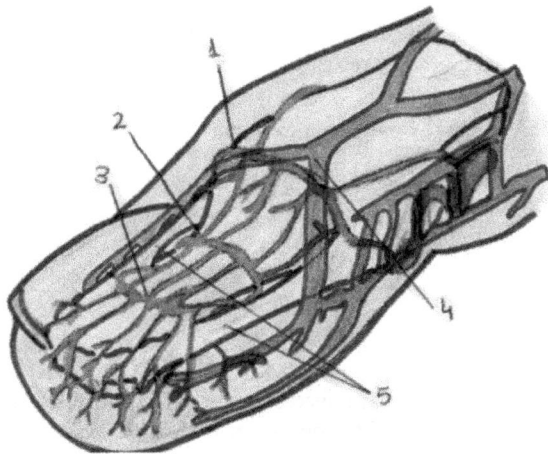

Figure 2.
Vascularity of the nail: 1. superficial arterial arcade; 2. proximal subungual arterial arcade system; 3. distal subungual arterial arcade system; 4. distal venous arch; and 5. lateral ligaments to flint.

3. Aims of nail treatment

Fingernails have an important role in hand function, because they protect the dorsal surface of the distal phalanges and increase sensitive of the fingertip. Furthermore, the nails facilitate the pinch of small objects and a cosmetic role. Hence, the aims of nail treatment are restoring a nail's length, morphology, and a normal appearance.

4. Principles of nail surgery

The nail trauma surgery can be do in the emergency department, but if the patient presents some digits with nail trauma or important lesions with a complex repair, we must think in an operative theater for do the treatment.

The patient should always be lying on a stretcher and good anesthesia is of paramount important. Any local anesthetic can be used (lidocaine, mepivacaine, etc.). We think that ropivacaine 1% is the election choice because have a long duration (8–12 h) and nail surgery usually is appreciated by patient as is often followed by intense pain. Technique of proximal digital anesthesia block make possible to do all types of nail surgery.

Except for subungual hematoma and nail avulsion, sterile prepping is a must for nail operations. Donning a sterile glove and cutting a tiny hole into the corresponding finger, which is then rolled back, not only gives a sterile file but also exsanguinates the finger and is an efficient tourniquet [2]. After realizing the tourniquet, bleeding is usually copious, and a thick padded dressing is necessary.

The major principles of repairs are the following:

- The nail bed is in direct relation to the periosteum of F3, a reduction defect and/or a prominence bone causes a deformation of the bed and, secondary form, of the nail sheet.

- The adhesion of the nail sheet is only possible if the reconstruction of the nail bed is perfect.

- The growth of the nail sheet is only possible from of the matrix, so that any injury of the matrix must be repaired carefully.

- Where possible, keep the nail sheet to replace it after the repair; failing that, a prosthesis can be used [3].

5. Material for nail treatment

It's important a sterile ambient, like any other surgical treatment. But it is almost always ambulatory surgery. Antibiotics are needed in most injuries and the use of magnification is essential for nail bed repair.

Very few special instruments are necessary for nail surgery. The suture material must be absorbable and of a small caliber. We use a Vicryl 6/0 for nail bed repair, and a non-absorbable monofilament for repair the surrounding soft tissue injuries and to fix the nail plate when we must remove it.

6. Nail trauma assessment

Fingertip and nail bed injuries are seen at all ages, with a peak incidence in 4–30 years old patients [4]. In the emergency department is important to detail in the clinical history the mechanism of injuries, the time it occurred, dominant hand, the patient's job and the context in which the trauma occurred to consider the possible contaminants of the wound.

Depending on the injury mechanism we will have to consider possible associated injuries. Fingertip injuries most frequently result from a crush injury, often from the hinge side of a door [5]. Approximately 50% of nail bed injuries presenting to hospital are associated with distal phalangeal fractures [6]. Simple radiographic (anteroposterior and lateral) is mandatory when a nail trauma is.

7. Treatment of nail injuries

7.1 Subungual hematoma

Nail bed is a highly vascular structure. If the nail is not broken with the trauma, blood collects beneath the nail and the pressure of which may cause pain. In these cases, it is a necessary treat. Drainage of the hematoma can be done by a paper clip heated or battery-powered ophthalmic cautery. Touch to nail at 90-degree angle over the central area of hematoma. The key of the treatment is to ensure that the hematoma is not older than 48 h and a round hole completely through the nail, which stay open to drain.

Once a hole is created it is expected that blood will drain out from the hematoma resolving most of the patient's pain. It may take more than one trephination to decompress the hematoma completely. Take care when advancing through the nail to avoid damage to the nail bed. Bandage site with sterile gauze in instruct patient to keep digit clean and dry.

If more than 50% of the nail bed is undermined by hematoma, the nail should be removed and explored the nail bed and the distal phalanx because can be affected.

7.2 Dislocation of the nail plate

These traumas occur when the mechanism of injury has a component of hyperflexion. The nail plate must be replaced in the nail fold. Before this, it is necessary

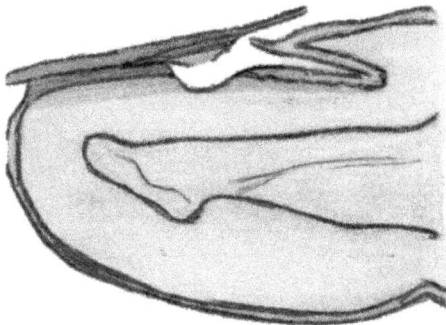

Figure 3.
Dislocation of the nail plate; with the reposition of the proximal nail plate, the nail bed avulsed is holding like a graft.

to verify the absence of any injury to the bed under local anesthesia. When the nail bed is injured, but it is a small fragment and it's adhered to the nail plate, with the reposition of the nail it is enough because it is like holding a graft (**Figure 3**).

A radiography is mandatory to ensure the absence of distal phalanx fracture because is often present. When there is a distal phalanx fracture associated, the nail plate reinstated and it is enough to stabilize the fracture, and no osteosynthesis or additional splinting is required. But generally, a distal phalanx fracture associated a dislocation of the nail base have a nail bed injury.

The nail plate is replaced into the nail fold to prevent scarring between the dorsal roof and the ventral floor. If more exposure of the nail fold is required, incisions are made at the proximal edge like **Figure 4** from the eponychium because are easier to approximate and cause less scarring than an incision made straight proximal.

7.3 Nail bed injuries and distal phalanx fracture

It is an injury similar than anterior apart, but the base of the nail remains in place. Classically, a fingertip crushed by the door. It is a frequent injuries of the nail unit and nail bed injuries are easily overlooked especially in children as they are less cooperative and more difficult to do an adequate inspection of the lesions [7].

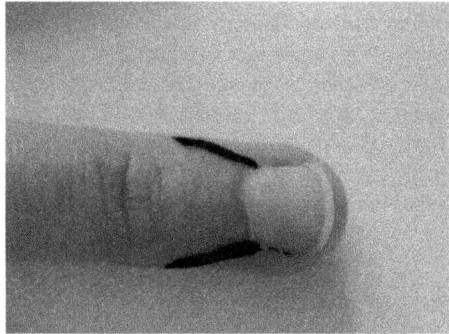

Figure 4.
Kanavel incisions.

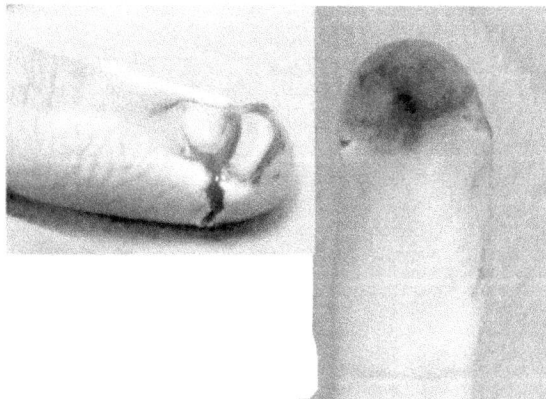

Figure 5.
A 20-year-old man with second finger entrapment of his right hand with a door. The wounds affect paronychium and the lateral edges of the pulp.

The impact of the nail complex results from palmar displacement of the distal fragment (**Figure 5**).

The proximal nail plate is gentle elevated. Care should be taken to elevate the nail plate without the nail bed and the other tissue. And the distal nail plate is elevating too. Now, the nail bed is explored, and irregularities of the edges may be trimmed into a straight line if it can be closed without tension. After the nail bed is approximated with an absorbable suture 6/0 or 7/0, the nail plate is replaced into the nail fold and held with 4/0 or 5/0 suture to hyponychium.

Approximately 50% of nail bed injuries have an associated fracture of the distal phalanx [8]. An associated fracture with a wound in the nail indicates a high energy trauma. The nail plate replaced serves as a splint, and usually osteosynthesis is not necessary. But an osteosynthesis by an axial wire is essential when the distal phalanx fragment is big, or the fracture is instable. A proper alignment of the bone fragments must be done because otherwise it may generate future nail deformities.

Figure 6 shows the case of a middle-aged woman with entrapment of the third finger of her left hand with the door of her vehicle. She had an associated fracture

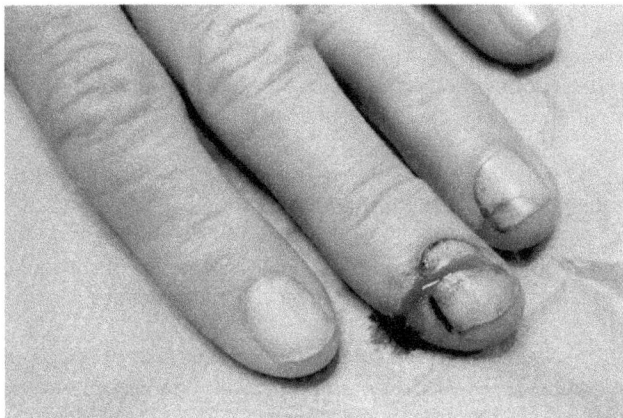

Figure 6.
Example of nail trauma in a woman.

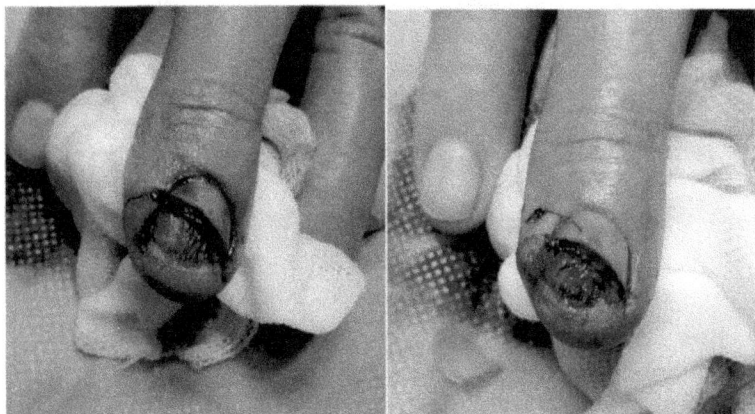

Figure 7.
Left: wound in the nail bed. Right: nail bed sutured.

of the distal phalanx. After elevated the nail plate, we observe a wound in the nail bed, which is approximated with an absorbable suture 6/0 (**Figure 7**). Then, the nail plate is again repositioned and fixed. The nail plate has a double function; protection of the nail bed repaired and like a splint for the fracture (**Figure 8**).

7.4 Crushing injuries

These types of injuries resulting from a wide area of force applied to the nail. This energy causes an explosive type of injury in the nail bed with many fragments (**Figure 9**). In this type of lesion, it is important that all fragments of the nail be attached to the periosteum. So that, when the nail plate is being raised, we must be careful in these. No fragments of nail bed should be debrided and discarded because it is extremely difficult to replace. Like the anterior apart, these fragments are approximated whit fine suture, and the nail plate or a synthetic substitute is used to mold the fragments prevent scaring.

7.5 Nail bed avulsions or tissue loss

Tissue lost affecting the distal half of the nail bed are more common than affecting the proximal half, because the distal end of the nail is more exposed to trauma. Many methods or treatment have been described, but still today it continues generating doubts about which is the best method to reposition the lost nail bed.

Depending on the size of the fragment of nail bed avulsed:

- Less than 1–2 mm, it can be replaced as accurately as possible with the nail plate and held in place with Steri-Strips or suture.

- Larger than 2 mm, the nail around the edge is removed of the nail bed and the fragment avulsed is suturing in their place, if it is possible.

Some authors consider the nail bed to have regenerative capacity and recommend, for limited tissue losses, promoting this healing by placement the nail plate or a substitute when the latter has been missed [3].

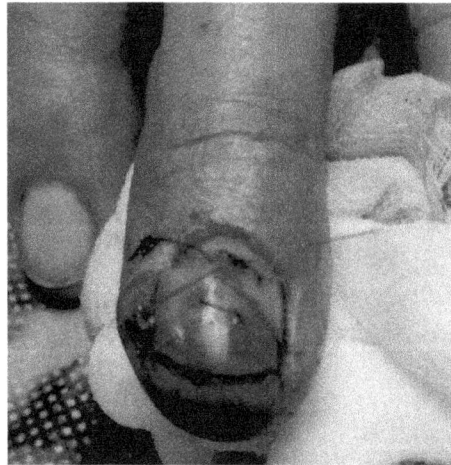

Figure 8.
Nail plate repositioned.

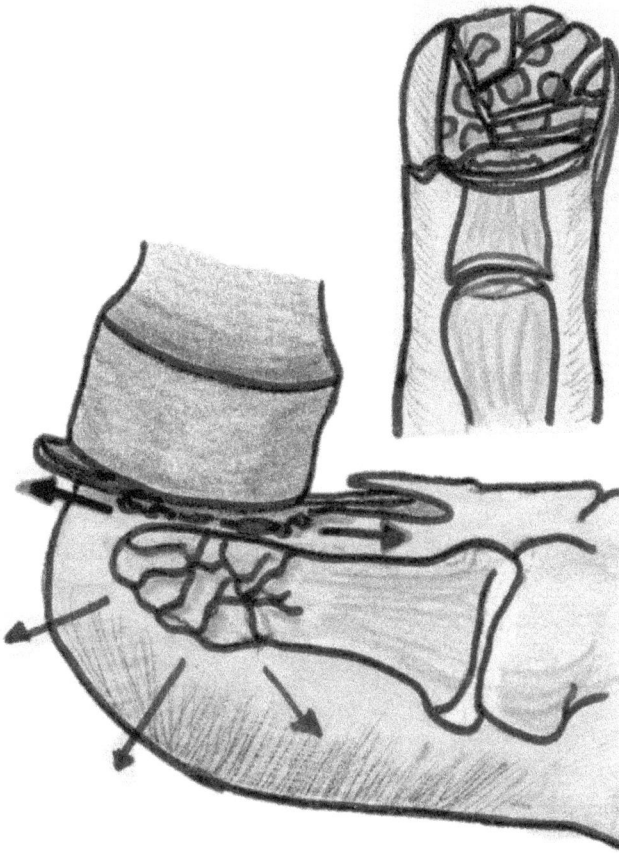

Figure 9.
Crushing injury of the nail.

When the fragment avulsed is missed, diverse treatments have been suggested, like skin grafts [9], reversal dermal grafts [10] or palatal mucosal grafts [11]. Even, porcine xenotransplants has been proposed . But we still have not found a histological tissue that can restore nail plate. So that, nail bed grafts are the best option actually, which can be full thickness grafts [12] or thin nail bed grafts [13, 14]. These techniques are highly specialized that must be performed by expert hand surgeons, so they are not of interest for this chapter.

8. Care after treatment

After performing the appropriate treatment based on the trauma presented by the patient, a cure of the injured finger should be made. The dressing chosen to perform the cure should be non-stick dressing (Vaseline) and must allow to leave free the proximal interphalangeal joint to avoid stiffness.

The first dressing change should be due in 48–72 h, to verify the absence of collection (hematoma, infection) and of pain.

The hand should be carried high with a sling. Analgesics are essential in 24–48 h and antibiotics may be necessary in some situations, especially in highly contaminated traumatism.

9. Conclusion

The pattern of fingernail injury depends in the energy and direction of trauma. Management of a fingernail injury should be selected based on injury type and extent and requires accurate knowledge of nail anatomy and physiology. An effective emergency treatment is mandatory to prevent secondary deformities and reduce the risk of secondary reconstruction of the nail bed, which often gives unpredictable results.

Conflict of interest

The author declares no conflicts of interest.

Author details

Rebeca Astorga Veganzones
University Hospital of Burgos, Burgos, Spain

*Address all correspondence to: rebecaastorga25@gmail.com

IntechOpen

References

[1] Patel L. Management of simple nail bed lacerations and subungual hematomas in the emergency department. Pediatric Emergency Care. 2014;**30**:742-745

[2] Hasegawa K et al. The microvasculature of the nail bed, nail matrix, and nail fold of a normal human fingertip. The Journal of Hand Surgery. 2001;**26**(2):283-290

[3] Ogunro EO. External fixation of injured nail bed with the INRO surgical nail splint. The Journal of Hand Surgery. 1989;**14**:236-241

[4] Nanninga GL et al. Case report of nail bed injury after blunt trauma; what lie beneath the nail? International Journal of Surgery Case Reports. 2015;**15**:133-136

[5] Yildirimer L et al. Experience of nail bed injuries at a tertiary hand trauma unit: A 12-month review and cost analysis. The Journal of Hand Surgery, European Volume. 2019;**44**(4):419-423

[6] Satku M, Puhaindran ME, Chong AK. Characteristics of fingertip injuries in children in Singapore. Hand Surgery. 2015;**20**:410-414

[7] Yorlets RR, Busa K, Eberlin KR, et al. Fingertip injuries in children: Epidemiology, financial burden, and implications for prevention. Hand (New York, N.Y.). 2017;**12**(4):342-347

[8] Zook EG, Guy RJ, Russell RC. A study of nail bed injuries. Causes, treatment and prognosis. The Journal of Hand Surgery. 1984;**9A**:247-252

[9] Flatt A. Nail bed injuries. British Journal of Plastic Surgery. 1956;**8**:38-43

[10] Clayburgh RH, Wood MB, Cooney WP 3rd. Nail bed repair and reconstruction by reverse dermal grafts. The Journal of Hand Surgery. 1983;**8**:594-598

[11] Fernandez-Mejia S, Dominguez-Cherit J, Pichardo-Velazquez P, Gonzalez-Olvera S. Treatment of nail bed defects with hard palate mucosal grafts. Journal of Cutaneous Medicine and Surgery. 2006;**12**:69-72

[12] Ersek RA, Gadaria U, Denton DR. Nail bed avulsions treated with porcine xenografts. The Journal of Hand Surgery. 1985;**10**:152-153

[13] Lazar A, Abimelec P, Dumontier C. Full thickness skin graft for nail unit reconstruction. Journal of Hand Surgery (British). 2005;**30**:194-198

[14] Matsuba HM, Spear SL. Delayed primary reconstruction of subtotal nail bed loss using a split-thickness nail bed graft on decorticated bone. Plastic and Reconstructive Surgery. 1988;**81**:440-443

www.ingramcontent.com/pod-product-compliance
Lightning Source LLC
Chambersburg PA
CBHW081234190326
41458CB00016B/5783